# Total Health Transformation

## Dr Danny Scahill DC

# Testimonials

"The improvements I've noticed since I began the course have been amazing, my life has completely reformed! Before I used to suffer with Irritable Bowel Syndrome (IBS) and I was totally exhausted all of the time, when I got home after work I would literally be ready for bed! I'm glad to say I now have easy comfortable digestion and renewed energy!

I started to notice boosts in energy within a few short days of starting Danny's Total Health Transformation Programme and then the benefits just kept on building and building after that really!"

**Ursula Crossan**
**– Recruitment Consultancy Business Owner**

"Before I met Danny Scahill, I had a major lack of energy in the afternoons which prevented me from working effectively. I wasn't exercising, and had previously quit the gym twice. I'm naturally slim so found it hard to keep the motivation to get fit.

I also suffered from lower back pain and sometimes had problems sleeping through the night.

After a few coaching sessions with Danny, on his Total Health Transformation programme, I started to make small but regular improvements to my life to help me feel and think better.

I joined a new gym, setting up a training regime that I could stick to, ensured that I walked at least 10,000 steps per day, booked onto classes to help my lower back, and drank sufficient water and my own healthy juices each day.

These changes have helped me to feel healthier, concentrate on my work throughout the day and sleep better at night.

I recommend Danny's coaching programme especially if you've struggled in the past to have a healthier lifestyle and want to make a positive difference to your health and well-being."

**Phil Hampton,**
**Managing Director at Cartoon Media Ltd**

"The improvements in my health and consequently my business have been outstanding and I have Dr. Danny to thank for that! I think this programme could benefit anyone but I've found business owners and entrepreneurs tend to be much more motivated to want to maximise their energy to improve their bottom line just like I did!

I was active in the whole process of transforming my health with the trainings; I wasn't just a guinea pig! I was educated about Eating Well, Moving Well and Thinking Well. I found the whole programme to be most educational and holistic – in the sense that I had never before considered restoring and balancing my mind-body in order to improve my business! I would recommend that anyone who wants to improve their overall health and the health of their business then have a Breakthrough Consultation with Dr. Danny – you won't regret it!"

**Dominique MacNally**
**– Graphic Design Company Director**

"Just under 6 months ago, life was more than a bit of a struggle! I had great difficulty in standing up from a chair, walking up stairs and riding my bike was just out of the question! It was impossible for me to do any physical tasks and our other hobby of ballroom dancing was being severely hampered! I had a lot of pain especially in my knees and I generally felt very run down and tired most of the time!

Now six months later – **WOW what a change!**

We've just come back from our holiday where we went on several bike rides, one being over 5 miles and the other one just less than 20 miles! Incredible! Thank you, Dr. Danny! My wife and I also went for walks along the beach, the longest being a 6-mile walk – something I could have only dreamed about 6 months ago!

Your Coaching Programme was very easy to follow and thanks to your very simple diet recommendations I've now lost over 3 stone in the last 3 months which is amazing! I've now got more energy than I've had in the last 25 years which is great because we have a very active retirement planned! I just wish I'd known about your programme sooner Danny!"

#### John Fisher – Retired Business Man

First published in United Kingdom in 2018 by Scahill Health & Wellness Ltd

ISBN 978-0-9945944-9-5

**Disclaimer**
All the information, techniques, skills and concepts contained within this publication are of the nature of general comment only, and are not in any way recommended as individual advice. The intent is to offer a variety of information to provide a wider range of choices now and in the future, recognising that we all have widely diverse circumstances and viewpoints. Should any reader choose to make use of the information herein, this is their decision, and the author and publisher/s do not assume any responsibilities whatsoever under any conditions or circumstances. The author does not take responsibility for the business, financial, personal or other success, results or fulfilment upon the readers' decision to use this information. It is recommended that the reader obtain their own independent advice.

# Foreword

Anyone who wants to succeed and thrive in life understands that taking care of your physical health is vital. How you feel, think and move in your body every day either limits your potential or unlocks it.

My first decade in business taught me this as I spent several years working myself into the ground until I was severely burned out. My performance and results – not to mention my ability to plan long-term success for my business – suffered as a result.

Today I know that every decision I make about the food I eat, the movement I make, how I use my time, and what I do to rejuvenate my body truly does define the type of life I will live and what I will achieve in that life.

Many people feel that taking care of their health is a cost on their time in a busy schedule. It's time for us to change this and, instead, respect every effort we make to take care of our bodies as what it truly is: an investment in an enriched future.

Danny both understands and practices the powerful principles that unlock sustainable wellbeing in the body. I know his holistic approach to health and healing has assisted many people to experience increased energy levels, prolonged vitality, and a better quality of life.

I hope you implement what he teaches in this book as I know it has the power to change your life from the inside-out.

With inspiration,

**Emily Gowor**
Author & Speaker

# Preface

My story really is a struggle against adversity; there are multiple occasions where I could reference that. When I was fifteen I experienced injuries to my shoulder and low back from lifting weights. I had to stop exercise overnight – and I was doing a lot of exercise at that time including football, kickboxing and karate too. Prior to this point I had never really known what stress was; never really experienced it because I was so fit and so healthy – and I had regular exercise as a release valve. I never really knew what it was until I had to stop exercising due to injury. Without regular exercise the stress built up in me like a pressure cooker and it just got too much for me. Fairly soon after I was forced to stop exercising and I ended up getting really depressed.

This didn't happen overnight; it happened gradually and it was at the time I was doing my GCSEs (the UK's equivalent of the high school diploma). So I was going through all of these different exams and I had a lot of course work to do. Things were just getting on top of me. I ended up getting really depressed — clinically depressed, in fact. When I look back at that time I don't wish ever to be there again. It was a horrible experience to become clinically depressed. It was at that time when I first began to learn of the link between exercising and good mental health.

Luckily enough, I was able to speak to my parents about it; I could tell them about it, express my fears and concerns. When I look back at that time and think about it, I can still remember the feeling of fear and anxiety in the pit of my stomach. It was such an emotional time. I wouldn't wish depression on my own worst enemy, I really wouldn't.

My parents spoke to my teachers; they then reassured me and my parents that as far as they were concerned I was doing well in class and I wasn't behind. I was up to date and everything was okay which was fantastic! I ended up passing every single exam — I got really good grades, passing all ten exams I then went on to do my A-levels, (the next stage between high school and university, if you are based outside the UK).

## WHO AM I?

Never in the whole of human history has there been a more urgent need to address the issues of deteriorating health and well-being. I believe that better nutrition, mindset, and exercise are essential ingredients for creating more motivation, energy and health, leading to the achievement of ultimate performance for business owners. I have been in the health arena for over half of my life and I've always been fascinated by what makes people healthy or not as the case may be. I believe it is very simple. It comes down to three things: eat, move and think on purpose.

Way back when I was fifteen years of age, I was very active, doing lots and lots of exercise, used to playing football at least twice a day. Being from Liverpool, football is like a religion really, to be fair. So we would play a lot of football when we were growing up. I also did lots of martial arts as well, including karate and also kickboxing, three or four times a week. So I was very active, very fit and very healthy.

I had a competition coming up, some kickboxing tournaments were just around the corner. When I was fifteen years of age I was only somewhere around 5-foot-1 or 5-foot-2, absolutely tiny. I'm not huge now to be honest with you, I'm only 5-foot-7, but I was tiny at that stage in my life I had these tournaments coming up and I decided, in my infinite wisdom, that I would get some weights for my birthday to get bigger and stronger for these tournaments. Many of the people I was coming up against were a lot bigger than me. So I started lifting weights against the advice of my dad, who said, "You're only going to get injured

Daniel, you're too young." I responded, "Dad, come on, it's my birthday, can you just get me the weights, please." So I got the weights. I didn't really know what I was doing. I lifted weights that were too heavy and had a poor training technique. To cut a long story short, I injured myself. And that was what ultimately led me down the route of becoming a chiropractor.

First of all I went to see a physiotherapist. Personally that didn't do anything; luckily, my mum had free health insurance for the whole family from the work that she was doing. It cost an absolute fortune but unfortunately did not help me at all. So the next thing I tried was osteopathy. I remember speaking to my mum and she says, "Why don't you go and see this osteopath that I've been seeing for a while. It's really helping me and I reckon it will help you." So I went to see the osteopath.

At that time I had applied to study law at university – ever since I was the age of four or five, believe it or not, I wanted to be a lawyer. Never met any kids that young since then who knew how to say the word 'barrister', let alone understood what it means! The reason that's relevant is because I went to the osteopath and found it really good; it started to help me, so I looked at what they were doing and I thought "That looks really interesting. And it looks like they can make a good living helping people get well." At that point, I was around about the age seventeen and I had already applied to do law. But once I realised I did not want to do law any more, I withdrew my application and applied instead to go to osteopathic college.

I continued to see the osteopath, did my A-levels and went to osteopathic college when I was eighteen. It was going to be either a four- or five-year course; however, four years into it, when I could almost see the finish line, the college closed down! As it happened, both professions – chiropractic and osteopathy – were getting regulated at that time and all part-time colleges got closed down: everything from that point on had to be full time on the undergraduate courses, whereas mine was part time. When I was training, from the age of eighteen to twenty-one, I worked full time as well as studying, so it was hard going.

When the college closed down, as you can imagine I was not happy! I was really upset for a short period of time. Then I realised: okay, I didn't have the whole university experience at osteopathic college, because I was working full time and studying. An osteopath mentor of mine asked "Why don't you become a chiropractor?" And that in itself was a revelation, because all the way through osteopathic college a lot of the tutors would say, "If you've got a patient you don't like and you don't want to see any more, send them to the chiropractor or the physio down the road!" (Further down the line, when I was in Chiropractic College, all of the teachers used to say,

"If you've got a patient you don't like, send them to the osteopath or the physio down the road.")

I applied to study chiropractic at university at what was then Glamorgan University in South Wales, at the Welsh Institute of Chiropractic (WIOC). I went for an interview, got accepted and trained for five years to become a Doctor of Chiropractic. That, in itself, was a big achievement: not many people finished that five-year course. 120 people started but fewer than 50 graduated. I worked hard through this long journey and, after nine years of training, eventually adjusted my first Chiropractic patient.

So there were one or two struggles with adversity along the way for me and that's part of what really led to me down this path towards where I am now. As well as being a practising Doctor of Chiropractic, I am also a Peak Performance Expert working with people like you. I work with business professionals and entrepreneurs to help transform energy and performance, so that they get to live the life and enjoy the business that they desire

As you can see I am extremely determined; once I set out to do something I don't stop until it's achieved. That really holds my patients and clients in good stead – when they work with me, I don't give up on them. We set out to do something and we achieve it. At the time of writing this book, I've done nine years of Chiropractic and Osteopathic training and have been in Chiropractic practice for over 10 years – so I'm very experienced in the health and wellness field.

Over the years many people have asked me to help with various things regarding their health. That might be to lose weight, to get fit or to get more energy. It all started to become apparent in my early stages of my chiropractic career that the vast majority of people who come in to my chiropractic centre do so because they're in pain or they have symptoms of some sort.

In a lot of ways, though, it's not usually the pain that they come in to get fixed. That's what they think at that time – but really, when it comes down to it, they're coming in to try and get that pain fixed so that they can get their 'desired outcome' so that they can get back to doing that desired thing, whatever that is. Whether that is the need to be free of pain, so that they can play with their kids, or that they can go for a run and compete in a marathon, or that they can be comfortable sitting down in their job. Whatever it is, it's usually because they want a desired result – not necessarily because they want to get free of pain.

It was when I began in Chiropractic practice that I realised there's more to this health thing than just getting people free of pain. It's very much about looking at the whole picture: getting things back into balance, facilitating people to be able to live the life that they want to, to be the most vibrant and the healthiest that they can be.

As I mentioned earlier I have been in this health arena, for over half my life now. I have many qualifications and experience that will help you get to where you want to go to, including the health and wellness-related experience in Chiropractic and also my work as an NLP practitioner and Peak Performance Coach. I've also completed numerous different training programmes in many different fields that will be able to assist you on your journey.

It saddens me to see so many people today not living to their peak potential in terms of their Health, Energy, and Vitality. If you're looking for a transformation in your health then you are in the right place and with the right information and guidance it's actually much easier than you think to achieve your desired outcome.

If you're a person who needs more energy, wants to lose weight, you're constantly stressed out and want to learn how to reduce stress then – Total Health Transformation is absolutely for you! I invite you to read on, absorb the information and most importantly implement the Total Health Transformation system and your world will change forever!

# Table of Contents

# Introduction

If you are suffering with any of these 3 three major issues: lack of energy, being chronically stressed out or suffering from unwanted weight gain, then you are out of balance and this book will show you the 3 step process to help you get back into balance and transform your health in the process. When your **exercise**, **nutrition** and **mindset** routines are out of balance, that's when you will likely suffer with low energy, chronic stress and unwanted weight gain

Business people tend to have less free time to take care of themselves; more pressures of running the business (or of staying employed) in a competitive economy. Many health treatments, fine though they are in principle, are just not practical for most people. So, if you can recognise any of these issues, or have been nodding and thinking how this applies to you - then this book is for you.

Let's explore the issue in more detail:

## Lack of energy:

Lack of energy is extremely common these days, due to the demands that people have on their body day to day; particularly on business owners, because they require a lot of energy to make a success of their business. Because they're not eating the right foods, they're not exercising correctly or doing the right strategies with regards to their mindset and so they are suffering with regards to their energy. So if you have a lack of energy and you are a business professional, then this book is for you as low energy leads to a lack of clarity, poor decision making and struggling to think quickly.

## Chronically stressed out:

People are stressed out of their minds at work these days. And it's only going to get worse as more and more is expected from people, whether they are running the business themselves or whether they're an entrepreneur within a business looking to breakaway to go out on their own. Stress is a huge problem and we hear people talk about this all of the time. It's across the media, it's in the newspapers, it's on the TV, and it's in the magazines.

Stress is the biggest killer in the 21st century. That's not to say it hasn't always been. It has, but it has become more and more mainstream. In the last ten years stress has become a massive buzzword within the general public. So, I will elaborate a lot more on what stress is, but with regards to this book and why you should read this book. If you are feeling stressed at work, then you need to read this book.

## Unwanted weight gain:

The third person for whom this book is for, is someone who has put on weight. Now it's more and more common these days to see people who have put on extra weight. Again because of what they eat, how they move and how they think. Eat well, move well, think well is absolutely essential if you want to get healthy and stay healthy and if you're not doing those three things correctly, then you're going to put weight on. Now, weight gain is a massive problem in the western world today and it's been getting worse year upon year for the last ten or even twenty years and that is largely because people are not eating, moving and thinking on purpose.

Weight gain is a huge problem, which started off twenty or thirty years ago, in America. I remember, when I was a child, going over to Florida to Disney World and we were astounded how overweight and indeed obese a huge percentage of people were over there. It was no surprise really when we saw the size of the meals that they were given; massive portions of the wrong foods. But people are eating the wrong foods today – and as we've noticed throughout history really, whatever happens in America tends to happen in the rest of the world. We're eating the same foods. So if you're doing the same thing, you're getting the same result. It's commonsense really.

## HOW THIS BOOK CAN HELP YOU

This book describes how my three-part system can help you overcome many problems, such as the following:

- Life's not fun, it's a struggle.
- I want to regain quality of thinking.
- I'm not sleeping very well.
- Exercise doesn't work for me, I don't enjoy it.
- I've got low energy, I'm exhausted.
- I lack motivation.
- I'm putting weight on and I don't know why.
- I lack self-worth.
- I'm not confident when I pitch for new business; I could do with a lot more confidence.
- I'm all over the place, I can't focus on things.

These are just some of the things that Total Health Transformation can and has addressed in many of my clients. These areas are problems that past and present clients started with when they began on the journey with me, through my Total Health Transformation programmes.

Here are, for example, some comments on specific issues:

- **Life's not fun, it's a struggle**

  Life shouldn't be a struggle, it should be fun. We really all deserve to be in the flow and doing what we love and just enjoying the process, enjoying the journey. My programmes can help you address and rebalance your health, mindset and your lifestyle.

- **I'm putting weight on and I don't know why**

  We need to eat on purpose, move on purpose and think on purpose if we want to be truly healthy. But if we're not eating the right things – or eating the wrong things at the wrong times – or we're not exercising or we are stressed out of our minds, then it's quite likely that we're going to put weight on. However, by addressing just a few small things, making a few small changes can make a drastic difference to your body, your life and your lifestyle.

- **Not being able to think clearly**

  That is something that is often easy to remedy with a few simple techniques to turn around, to give you clarity of thought and calm and peace of mind.

- **Not sleeping very well**

  What we do is address what's causing these sleeping issues. If we can help you get to the root cause of the problem and address that head on, you'll be able to sleep like a baby once again.

- **Exercise doesn't work for me**

  Well the thing is, exercise will work as part of a healthy balanced diet. The moving on purpose, on its own, without the thinking or the eating on purpose, is not going to achieve the desired result. It's part of the triad of health, it doesn't stand alone, it stands next to its peers, if you like: eating and thinking on purpose. The key, really, for any exercise is that you need to enjoy it. So pick an exercise you enjoy, otherwise you're not going to stick it out. It's not rocket science.

- **Low energy and exhaustion**

  This is generally easy to rectify. We do that by analysing everything that you do with regards to what you eat, how you move and how you think. The same goes for weight gain: analysing everything and then making the required recommendations – and holding you accountable to ensure you achieve the desired outcomes.

- **Lack of motivation**

  We all deserve to love what we do. If we do not love what we do, then we will naturally lack motivation. We need to find a big reason why we do what we do. What is it that gets you up in the morning, what's your purpose? On our Total Health Transformation programmes, we drill down and find out what your values are, what your purpose is, what you are here for. We reset that compass to drive you towards your goals, dreams and desires at lightning speed.

Over the years many people have asked me to help with various things regarding their health. That might be to lose weight, to get fit or to get more energy. You know, it all started to become apparent in my early stages of my chiropractic career that the vast majority of people who come in to my chiropractic practice do so because they're in pain or they have symptoms of some sort.

In a lot of ways, though, it's not usually the pain that they come in to get fixed. That's what they think at that time – but really, when it comes down to it, they're coming in to try and get that pain fixed so that they can get their 'desired outcome' so that they can get back to doing that desired thing, whatever that is. Whether that is the need to be free of pain, so that they can play with their kids, or that they can go for a run and compete in a marathon, or that they can be comfortable sitting down in their job. Whatever it is, it's usually because they want a desired result – not necessarily because they want to get free of pain.

It was when I began in Chiropractic practice that I realised there's more to this health thing than just getting people free of pain. It's very much about looking at the whole picture: getting things back into balance, facilitating people to be able to live the life that they want to, to be the most vibrant and the healthiest that they can be.

If you're a person who needs more energy, if you're a person who wants to lose weight, if you're a person who is constantly stressed out and needs to learn and wants to learn how to reduce stress, manage stress, and eradicate stress in some cases, then Total Health Transformation is absolutely for you.

# PART 1:
# EAT ON PURPOSE

# Chapter 1:
# Improve Your Health

Everyone wants to be healthy, what are some of the some of the signs that you're not healthy though?

## PROBLEMS OF POOR HEALTH

Have you ever stopped to think why people have problems? There are, inevitably, a host of reasons, but when you stop to analyse them they almost invariably come down to one of three key areas. People suffer from poor health because they are:

- **Demotivated**
- **Lacking energy**
- **Suffering from poor health**

This is especially common in business owners, as they are trying to juggle so many different things in their life – their business, themselves, their family and so on.

When somebody's health suffers, they are much more likely to take time off work. When you're the business owner, particularly if it's a small business, taking time out of the business means, generally, there's no money coming in. That naturally, massively increases stress levels. When health suffers as a result of poor performance; due to a lack of motivation, lack of energy or otherwise: people find themselves unable to cope with day-to-day life, running their business or looking after their families. And, following the vicious circle nature of the preceding problems, this inability to cope further exacerbates stress levels – which further compound the problem.

How Does Your Health stack up? Rate Your Current Health Score Below:

| Area | Out of 10 (10 Being Amazing!) |
|---|---|
| Motivation | |
| Energy Level | |
| General Health | |

A total health score of 30 is the aim here. Look at each section individually out of 10 and then collectively the total score out of 30. This will give you an indication of what area/s to address first

- A individual section score of less than 5 is critical and needs attention immediately to rectify it

- A total health score of 15 or less is critical and needs attention immediately to rectify it

## MANAGING POOR HEALTH

At the end of the day, nearly all of these problems arise because people do not focus on the triad of health: mindset, nutrition and exercise. Simply put, the problems of demotivation, poor energy and ultimately poor health result from this triad being out of balance. These elements are all intimately connected e.g. if we don't eat well, we won't have the right fuel to be able to exercise effectively and it we don't exercise regularly this will in turn increase stress levels which will have a negative impact on your mindset.

That's where the Total Health Transformation programmes proven system comes into play, so before we consider what causes somebody to have poor health, we have to go back to basics and ask ourselves what we mean by this word: health. If we don't understand what it is, there's little chance of improving it! This is similar to a point made later in the book: if you can't assess something, you can't modify it.

- **Defining health**
  Health is a state of complete physical, mental, and social wellbeing and not merely the absence of disease, illness, or infirmity. That is the World Health Organisation definition of health and it's one we subscribe to as Chiropractors and very much so in my role as a Peak Performance Expert as well.

To expand on that though, health is more than just feeling good (which is important) it's about being able to function at your best every day in every way. That is to function at 100% physically, emotionally and spiritually so this obviously will include being happy and fulfilled in your life and your work.

## EAT ON PURPOSE

Optimum nutrition is crucial to good health. Poor nutrition has a massive impact on your levels of motivation, energy and, obviously, your health. The old computing adage of 'garbage in, garbage out' is true – particularly when we look at nutrition. When you focus on nutrition in your life, it is really important that you put the right fuel into your body if you expect it to function at its best. As business owners, we all want to focus on performing at our best to get the most out of business, and thus to be able to have the lifestyle that we desire. When using any machine, if you expect it to perform at its best, you've got to put in quality fuel and servicing to get fantastic results; that's what we are looking for when we look to *Eat on Purpose*.

In the western world, people consume an acidic diet, one that's full of acid-producing food and drink. Refined carbohydrates are a big problem: they are broken down into strong acids, which can lead to lots of different health risks.

An acidic diet is very closely linked to lots of health problems and diseases. Just a few of these diseases would include the risk of coronary heart disease, diabetes, cancer and stroke. It's very important that our bodies are alkaline as opposed to acidic; more specifically, metabolically alkaline as opposed to acidic. A big issue that people in the western world have is that we consume dead nutrient-deficient foods.

That plays a big part in the fact that lots of people out there – maybe yourself included – are demotivated, lack energy and have poor health. There needs to be a focus on eating more live foods, and an increased focus on eating more organic fruit and veg. Another thing that would dramatically increase your body's performance is to significantly increase your intake of water. All of these factors will be covered in detail in later chapters.

## IMPLEMENTING *TOTAL HEALTH TRANSFORMATION NUTRITION*

A concept that needs to be understood is the acid-alkaline balance with regards to your nutrition and performance if you are intending on improving your motivation, energy and your health in your life and your business.

### What is the acid-alkaline balance?

You may have encountered (and remembered?) the pH scale chart (also known as the acid/alkaline chart, shown here at Figure 1) from school. Substances are listed in their order of acidity, (referred to as pH), ranging from 0 through to 14.

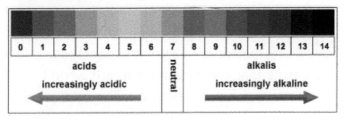

Figure 1: Summary Acid/Alkaline Chart

A modified chart, Figure 2, shows foodstuffs and their acidity rating. On the far left is pH1 - strong acid; in the middle is 7, which is pH neutral, and on the far right is pH 14 Strong Alkaline.

The middle is pH neutral, a value of 7 (7.34 is the pH of water). What is the significance of this with regard to what you eat? Here's an example for you and it's one of the most heavily consumed food groups around the world - dairy products. This will give you some indication as to how acidic the western diet is. It is extremely acid forming and this in itself causes a lot of potential health problems.

When you drink milk and your body breaks it down, milk is broken down into strong acid. This has lots of consequences within your body, simply because your body is not supposed to be acidic; rather, it is supposed to be slightly alkaline. There is only one place in your body that should be acidic and

| Acid | Healthy Body pH Range | Alkaline |
| --- | --- | --- |
| < 5.0  5.0  5.5 | 6.0  6.5  7.0  7.5  8.0 | 8.5  9.0  9.5+ |

| Most Acid | Acid | Lowest Acid | FOOD CATEGORY | Lowest Alkaline | Alkaline | Most Alkaline |
| --- | --- | --- | --- | --- | --- | --- |
| NutraSweet, Equal, Aspartame, Sweet 'N Low | White Sugar, Brown Sugar | Processed Honey, Molasses | SWEETENERS | Raw Honey, Raw Sugar | Maple Syrup, Rice Syrup | Stevia |
| Blueberries, Cranberries, Prunes | Sour Cherries, Rhubarb | Plums, Processed Fruit Juices | FRUITS | Oranges, Bananas, Cherries, Pineapple, Peaches, Avocados | Dates, Figs, Melons, Grapes, Papaya, Kiwi, Berries, Apples, Pears, Raisins | Lemons, Watermelon, Limes, Grapefruit, Mangoes, Papayas |
| Chocolate | Potatoes (without skins), Pinto Beans, Navy Beans, Lima Beans | Cooked Spinach, Kidney Beans, String Beans | BEANS VEGETABLES LEGUMES | Carrots, Tomatoes, Fresh Corn, Mushrooms, Cabbage, Peas, Potato Skins, Olives, Soybeans, Tofu | Okra, Squash, Green Beans, Beets, Celery, Lettuce, Zucchini, Sweet Potato, Carob | Asparagus, Onions, Vegetable Juices, Parsley, Raw Spinach, Broccoli, Garlic |
| Peanuts, Walnuts | Pecans, Cashews | Pumpkin Seeds, Sunflower Seeds | NUTS SEEDS | Chestnuts | Almonds | |
| | | Corn Oil | OILS | Canola Oil | Flax Seed Oil | Olive Oil |
| Wheat, White Flour, Pastries, Pasta | White Rice, Corn, Buckwheat, Oats, Rye | Sprouted Wheat Bread, Spelt, Brown Rice | GRAINS CEREALS | Amaranth, Millet, Wild Rice, Quinoa | | |
| Beef, Pork, Shellfish | Turkey, Chicken, Lamb | Venison, Cold Water Fish | MEATS | | | |
| Cheese, Homogenized Milk, Ice Cream | Raw Milk | Eggs, Butter, Yogurt, Buttermilk, Cottage Cheese | EGGS DAIRY | Soy Cheese, Soy Milk, Goat Milk, Goat Cheese, Whey | Breast Milk | |
| Beer, Soft Drinks | Coffee | Tea | BEVERAGES | Ginger Tea | Green Tea | Herb Teas, Lemon Water |

Figure 2: Acid Base Diagram

that would be your stomach. Nowhere else in your body should be acidic, but when you consume acid-forming products, in this case dairy products, then your body has to neutralise that acid: for survival, to the detriment of everything else.

The body has two ways of neutralising excess acid. Method number one is to take calcium out of the bone, and method number two is to take magnesium out of the muscles, your blood vessels and tissues. Both of these factors have a massive negative consequence; when calcium is regularly removed from bone that ultimately leads to osteoporosis. When magnesium is taken out of muscles and connective tissues, that leads to sore and tight muscles and muscle spasms. More crucially, if you take magnesium out of blood vessels it makes them constrict – and when blood vessels constrict, your blood pressure goes up. So high blood pressure is a direct consequence of an acidic diet.

There are therefore massive consequences to having a diet that is metabolically acidic (acid forming); dairy products are one of the foods that you'll see on the acid-alkaline chart that fit into this category. Generally speaking, strongly acidic foods dominate most of our Western diet.

All meat is acid forming (red meat more so than others) and dairy products also: you've got milk, cheese, butter and all derivatives thereof. Coffee, tea, soft drinks and alcohol are all strongly metabolically acidic; all of the refined carbohydrates are acidic forming – and refined carbs are also heavily consumed in the Western diet.

Look on the right side of the chart, and you'll be able to see that all the *alkaline*-forming foods are predominantly vegetables and fruit. I'm sure it's no surprise to you to find that vegetables and fruits are very high in vitamins, minerals and nutrients – but most people in the west don't consume anywhere near enough fruits and veg. When you have a plate of food, you should ensure that 70-80% of it is on the alkaline side and 20-30% of it is on the acid-forming side.

You don't need to completely cut out anything that's acid forming; you just need to be sensible and have things in the correct proportions: 80/20, ideally. So, now that you know this information, exactly what are you going to do with it? Did you know that 'to know and not do is to not know!'. The key is to take action...

We have just scratched the surface when we talk about implementing **Total Health Transformation**

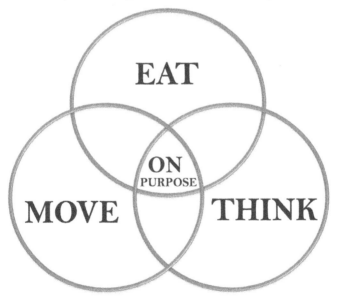

Figure 3 – The Total Health Transformation Trinity

***Nutrition***. We have so much more to cover later in this book – for example, the importance of water and how whatever you have been taught about water is wrong! I'll also be covering how to make the healthiest and most nutritious fresh juices, smoothies and soups – and much more!

## CHOOSING THE RIGHT FOODS FOR ENERGY AND PERFORMANCE

There are many symptoms of poor performance; three common ones that we're going to focus on in this chapter are:

- **Being stressed out and exhausted**
- **Weight gain**
- **Poor concentration**

All of the above are symptoms of being in, or experiencing, the stress response. You may have heard people talk about the 'fight or flight' response. If you think back to hunter-gatherer times, the males would go out hunting; if a tiger spotted them, the stress response ('fight or flight') would trigger in the body. This gives the person a 'rush' of adrenaline and also enough energy to do one of two things: either face the animal or enemy (fight) or run away (flight).

Typically when this stress response triggers in the body, running away will burn off the different adrenaline and stress hormones that get released into the body;

those chemicals are now not going to be harmful to the person's body. However, if we fast forward to the western world and society of today, our genes have not changed – yet the stress response still happens in the same way. What has changed is that we have very different environments and stimuli to contend with.

For example, if you're stressed out in work in your office (maybe you don't get on with your boss; or your boss, client, customer or supplier is having a go at you or you're just stressed out for one reason or another) the stress response still happens in your body – even if you're simply sat at your computer. The main difference compared to our ancestors is that we (usually) don't engage in any heavy physical fight-or-flight activity, so you don't get to burn off all of the different stress hormones. In today's sedentary lifestyle all the stress hormones stay in the body – where they cause lots of damage to the body by way of tissue damage and tissue death.

When we talk about the stress response, some of the symptoms that it will cause are; becoming chronically stressed out and exhausted, weight gain and poor concentration. So let's have a look at how that happens.

## Stress and exhaustion

In today's western world people, are constantly in a stress response, never really switching off. One of the aspects of modern life that has really speeded up the pace of life is technology. We live in a time when there are increasing demands on our time – both work and home. We're constantly available; almost everyone has a mobile phone and most have access to the internet on their phones. Social media makes us contactable 24/7, and we get countless emails or cold-calling phone calls every day.

Instant response is expected – or people feel under pressure to respond almost instantly. All of this builds on and compounds the stress response that's happening within the body, engendering a feeling of being out of control, of not being as responsive as your friend or co-worker.

## Weight gain

When one is chronically stressed out and exhausted, ultimately that's going to lead to weight gain. How does this happen? When we're constantly stressed out and exhausted we often grab unhealthy snacks for a quick fix, a quick boost of energy. Typically, when people snack on these unhealthy items, they are empty carbs: refined carbohydrates.

When you eat refined carbohydrates and you've got high stress (and you're not exercising as much as you should do) that causes weight gain; this vicious circle perpetuates poor concentration. All of these poor habits that we've talked about feed each other and that further compounds the problem.

## Poor concentration

When all the stress hormones enter into the bloodstream (because you generated increased feelings of stress, fear, anxiety and depression) that also has another effect on your body. It decreases your short-term memory, your ability to concentrate and your ability to learn. It also causes an increased sensitivity of the body's other sensory systems, especially those concerning pain and emotions.

# FOOD CHOICES

## What are the right foods?

Different gurus or health authorities have different opinions – and that further confuses the general public! Ideas seem to fall out of fashion; yesterday's bad guy is today's saviour. One expert tells me one thing, whereas another will tell us something completely different.

Let me give you my take on what good nutrition is – and what it is not. My views on this have changed over the years. I apply the 80/20 rule throughout life; right now we're talking about foods, though, so my approach is based on an 80% whole-food, plant-based diet and 20% not. I use organic meat, grass-fed and locally sourced. I also have several vegan days each week.

So, what foods are the right foods? You hear people talk about 'five a day' as being ideal, but the reality is that five pieces of fruit and vegetables per day should be regarded as an absolute minimum. The reality is that it's extremely easy to get far more than the five pieces of fruit and veg per day: you can do that by making things like regular smoothies, juicing or different soups. It is really easy to do, and these different strategies make it much easier.

Although you hear people talk about 'fruit and vegetables', you should think of it more as 'vegetables and fruit'. What do I mean by that? You'll focus on having a lot more vegetables than you do fruits. Although they're both important, vegetables will give you far more nutrition than the fruits – and without the sugars as well, which is key.

## Healthy fats

Over the years, there has been lots of media confusion around fat. Fat has been vilified. There are good fats and bad fats. The mass media over the past three or four decades has made fat the enemy; a low fat industry formed and lots of different low fat foods, low fat diets and stuff like that to get people to cut down their fat intake. Big companies could now market their products as 'low fat this, low fat the other'. The reality of the situation, however, is that it's not *fat* that makes people fat, it's *refined carbohydrates*: refined sugars, white sugars. These are the things that make somebody overweight. Just keep in your mind the simple fact: it is not fat that makes people fat.

Essentially, it is sugar that makes people fat. You will have noticed that almost anything that is low fat is high in sugars. So beware, beware indeed! There are healthy fats, the essential fatty acids. They're called 'essentials' because you need to have them in your diet: your body will not produce them. An example would be Omega 3 oils, which you've undoubtedly heard about and which you can get from many different sources.

Sources of Omega 3 can be fish oil, seeds and nuts – for example, flax seeds, sunflower seeds, pumpkin seeds or sesame seeds. These are all good sources of Omega 3 oils. You can also get mixed milled seeds, which are really handy because you can put them into smoothies, salads or stir fries. Another great source of Omega 3 oils is avocado, which is very high in the Omega 3s and other essential fatty acids and proteins. Because of its high fat content avocado has been vilified as being high fat when the reality is that it's extremely good for you.

## Organic produce

Buying organic fruits, vegetables and meat is far more affordable than people think. Historically, organic food has been more expensive than non-organic food but think about it logically. Would you choose to knowingly eat fruit and veg that is not organic, that has been heavily sprayed with pesticides, herbicides, fungicides – or would you rather eat fruit and veg that's not being sprayed by any of the above. Organic food is going to have far more nutrition in it as a result. With regards to organic produce, always do your best to make sure that you source it locally; there are lots of different companies that deliver boxes – fruit and veg boxes and meat boxes – each week, or you can go to farmers' markets and source it direct. One company I use is Abel & Cole (http:// www.abelandcole.co.uk/) who drop off fruit and veg boxes to the door once a week.

A great variety of organic food – fruit, veg and meat – is on offer from the major supermarkets. However, much of it is sourced from abroad, meaning it's going to have a lower nutritional content than if it were sourced locally. For example, think about certain fruit that you might get from the supermarket: it might say 'organic' on the label, but if it comes from Brazil, for example, it takes up to several weeks to come by ship. In the process of transit it's going to lose quite a lot of the nutrition, so make sure you source organically and source locally – so that the nutritional content of the food that you're eating is as high as possible. When you source organic food from local farmers' markets or companies as I mentioned, you really can taste the difference compared to the organic food from the supermarket – the difference can be phenomenal.

It really is a good idea to start to eat less meat; simply reduce the amount you eat. I say this from experience because, from a very young age, I have always really enjoyed meat. I still do today, but when I eat meat today I eat organic. If I'm buying it myself I always choose local organic grass-fed; when going out for a meal it can be more difficult, unless you're at an organic restaurant.

## FOOD MYTHS – AND WHAT TO AVOID

There are various different food groups that it's a good idea to limit your intake of – or reduce, or even eliminate. Before we go into different groups of food, let's look back to Figure 2 from the previous chapter – the acid/alkaline chart. Essentially what this refers to is the way the food that you eat is metabolised. Before you ingest it, what is the food? Is it acidic or is it alkaline? When you digest the food, what is it metabolised (broken down) into? Let's look at lemons and limes as an example: before you eat them they are extremely acidic – but after the body metabolises them and breaks them down they actually take form of alkaline items.

Another example is dairy products: before you drink milk, it's actually alkaline; when the body metabolises it and breaks it down, it becomes far more acidic – so we can say it's metabolically acidic. The significance of this is that, no matter what you eat and what you drink, your body will always – to the detriment of everything else – bring the pH of your blood chemistry and your body chemistry back towards pH neutral, which is around about 7-7.34 on the pH scale.

If you remember the acid/alkaline chart, very strong acid is shown on the far left, pH 1; very strong alkaline is shown on the far right, pH 14. pH 7 is pH neutral and is in the middle. Looking again at dairy products, you can see your body metabolises the dairy product into strong acid – but there's only one place in your body that is supposed to be acidic, and that area is the stomach. Everywhere else should be slightly alkaline.

Your brain tells your body it's got to get back towards pH neutral, as it has become acidic. (If it stayed in a state of acidity anywhere other than the stomach then this would give rise to a range of problems...) The body therefore has very strict objectives to get back to pH neutral as quickly as possible, and it does this in, primarily, two ways. Acid can be neutralised by going to the bone and taking calcium out of the bone. But if you take calcium out of the bone what happens? Yes, you guessed it, the bone gets weaker, allowing you to break bones much more easily. This eventually leads to osteoporosis.

The other thing that the body does, after it's taken calcium out of the bone, is to take magnesium out of the muscles and the blood vessels. Magnesium has many different functions, but the one we focus on here is that it relaxes muscles and it relaxes tissue. If you reduce the magnesium content it's going to make the muscles tight and contracted. Worse, if you take magnesium out, it's going to cause blood vessels to constrict – and if this happens blood pressure goes up, which can be extremely dangerous.

One group of food that is quite new, relatively speaking, is wheat-related products, wheat and gluten.

For many people the human body has not yet adapted to being able to digest wheat and gluten and to manage refined carbohydrates. Refined carbs and grains are quickly broken down and converted into glucose in the body; any unused blood sugar is then converted to, and stored as, fat – which ultimately leads to weight gain. I have a question for you: How do farmers fatten a cow? They feed it grain! I have news for you – it's the same for humans as well!

# TOTAL HEALTH TRANSFORMATION - CASE STUDY

"On our first, initial consultation, I was as scatty as anything, lacked focus, I was suffering with anxiety and panic attacks, I was overweight, couldn't sleep at night and as a result I was exhausted and pretty much burnt out to be honest.

Having now been through the Total Health Transformation programme I've got my drive back, my ambition has returned. My positive mental attitude has come back which is great! Before your programme, I was very, very lost. I was overwhelmed by absolutely everything whereas now I'm a lot calmer and focused.

I used to juice when I was a lot younger, you got me back into doing juicing and that had a profound effect on many levels for me on how energetic I am and how much more focused I became mentally.

Now it's like I'm obsessed, now my body only wants whole foods and nutritionally dense food. It rejects sugar —I was totally addicted to sugar before, anything sweet and I was there!

Now it's not even a case of, "Oh, I can't have that sweet treat." I don't even desire it, want it or crave it! Like you said on the programme Dr Danny, "focus on adding in good nutrition and eventually there will be no room or desire for the bad stuff and it just falls away!"

To say that the **Total Health Transformation** programme has been life changing is a huge understatement! Do it, you'll never look back and you'll never regret it. If you're looking to spend your money on anything and get a massive return on your investment, this is it. You will get a lifetime return on investment."

*Dee Patel – Business Development Consultant*

# RECIPES FOR SUCCESS

## How to select

Over the last few years I have been moving towards a whole-food plant-based diet, which is essentially a healthy vegan lifestyle. I look to follow a plant-based diet as closely as I can. I have to be honest though: as a meat eater every day for approximately the first 35 years of my life, it has been a huge challenge for me! (A whole-food plant-based diet is sometimes also referred to as an alkaline diet, just to confuse things even more...)

I currently aim to follow the 80/20 principle with my nutrition; this means that 80% of food and drink I consume are alkaline-forming foods and up to 20% are acid-forming food and drink. When I do consume meat, I make sure it is free range, organic and grass fed. I have 2-3 vegan days per week where I don't eat any meat or fish at all – and I don't eat eggs or dairy at all, in case you were wondering...

If you are just starting out on your journey though, I appreciate it can be quite daunting so my best advice is to take baby steps and implement things gradually rather than making big changes all at once. If you currently eat meat with most meals then you could start your journey by having one plant based meal per day or even every other day to begin with because every little helps!

When cattle is grass-fed and organic as it should be, the meat will naturally contain Omega 3 oils which, as we have indicated, are very good for your brain, heart and many other systems in your body. Omega 3 oils are healthy fatty acids that are also a natural anti-inflammatory in nature. By contrast, cattle that is grain-fed, non-organic and laden with antibiotics and growth hormones are devoid of any Omega 3 – and very high in Omega 6, which is inflammatory in nature.

## How to prepare

Eat raw foods (fruit, vegetables, nuts, seeds, etc.) as much as possible, as the process of cooking takes some of the nutrition out. If you must cook vegetables, then lightly steam them rather than boil them – steaming will retain more of the nutrition.

A blender is a fantastic piece of equipment to have in your kitchen. They are great for making healthy smoothies and healthy wholesome soups too! I have found a food processor invaluable in the past few years; they are so versatile and save so much time and effort when preparing meals.

# QUICK AND EASY RECIPES

## Breakfast Smoothie*

½ cup of organic raspberries or mixed berries (fresh or frozen)

½ organic cucumber

2 medium / large organic carrots

1 teaspoon of chia seeds soaked in 250ml high quality filtered water

1-2 sticks of celery

500ml of high quality filtered water

## Optional extras

1 apple

½ avocado

Note that all fruit and vegetables need washing before consuming.

I use a 1200w Duronic high powered blender, which can blend pretty much anything!

* You can have your smoothies any time, I just prefer them for breakfast or lunch.

## **Method**

- Pour 500ml filtered water into the blender

- Soak the chia seeds in 250ml of filtered water in a glass for 5 mins, stirring it every 60 seconds

- Roughly chop the cucumber and add to the blender. Peel and roughly chop the carrots and add to blender and blend.

- Add the ½ cup of berries and blend until smooth.

- Extra options: Core and chop the apple and blend.

- Mash up and add the ½ avocado; blend all until smooth

- Add more water if required. Serve and enjoy!

# LUNCH OR DINNER OPTIONS

## Cannellini Bean and Kale Stew / Soup

1 tablespoon olive oil

4 cloves of finely chopped garlic

1 medium onion finely chopped

150g raw kale, washed and well chopped

1 courgette chopped

1 400g tin cannellini beans, well rinsed

2 fresh tomatoes cut into 8s

1 teaspoon Italian herb seasoning

Squeeze of lemon juice

up to 500ml vegetable stock

Salt and pepper

## Method

- Heat the olive oil and sauté the onion until soft.
- Add the garlic and fry for a minute or so – don't let it brown.
- Add the kale and sauté until wilted.
- Add courgette and sauté for a couple of minutes.

- Add two-thirds of the beans, tomatoes, herbs and seasoning and stir well.

- Add stock (200ml for stew, 350ml for soup); cover and simmer for 5 minutes.

- Meanwhile put the remaining beans and a little stock into a blender and blitz until smooth.

- Stir into the simmering pan – this makes the sauce creamy.

- Continue to simmer for another 15 minutes or so, adding more stock if you need to.

- Turn off the heat and squeeze in the lemon juice.

- Serve over rice if it's a stew.

## **Notes**

You can use any greens (such as spring greens, leafy cabbage etc) instead of kale, depending on what's available. You could change this into a more Asian-inspired dish by using fresh or frozen edamame beans, and ginger and lemon grass instead of Italian herbs. Season well to taste.

*Above recipe included with permission from Karen Lee of the Sensitive Foodie Kitchen.*

## **Millet and Beetroot Balls**

½ cup millet

Vegetable stock/bouillon

bay leaf

3 medium sized carrots, grated

1 medium beetroot, grated

1 small red onion, grated

3 cloves roasted garlic

Italian herbs

garlic powder

fresh parsley

salt and pepper

3-4 heaped tablespoons gram/chickpea flour

## **Method**

- Cook the millet some time before you want to make your balls, to give it time to cool.

- Put the millet in a dry frying pan and toast over a medium heat until you smell a toasted aroma.

- Pour into a saucepan and cover with ½ cup of water, sprinkle of bouillon and a large bay leaf.

- Cover and bring to the boil.

- Once boiling, reduce heat right down and cook for 15 minutes or so until the water has been absorbed.

- Turn off the heat and leave to cook in the steam for a few minutes.

- Transfer to a bowl to cool, as you don't want it too mushy. Remove bay leaf.

- Add carrot, beetroot, onion, garlic, herbs, garlic powder and parsley to the millet and stir well to combine.

- Sprinkle over 3 spoons of gram flour and stir well.

- The mixture should start sticking together when pressed between your fingers.

- Add more flour if needed, and season with salt and pepper.

- Once everything is combined, take a large tablespoon of mixture and press firmly to form a tennis-ball-sized lump.

- Place on a lightly greased baking tray and repeat until all the mixture is used up.

- Bake in the oven at 180° for 20 minutes, then turn the balls over and bake for another 15 minutes or so until crunchy on the outside.

- Serve with a sauce of your choice.

*Above recipe included with permission from Karen Lee of the Sensitive Foodie Kitchen.*

## **Chicken / Vegetable Stir-fry (Serves 2-3 People)**

1 large white onion

3 cloves of garlic

1 thumb of ginger

2 organic chicken breasts (obviously not in the veggie version!)

2 carrots

Salt and pepper

Half to a whole courgette

4-5 tablespoons of Chinese soy sauce (low sugar)

½ cup of brown rice per person

Organic coconut oil or sunflower oil to cook

## **Method**

- Wash all the vegetables
- Peel and chop the carrots and the onion. Roughly chop the courgette.
- Peel and finely chop the garlic and ginger
- Bring a saucepan of water to the boil and boil the brown rice for about 20 mins
- Heat the oil in a wok and add the garlic and ginger and lightly brown
- Unless making the vegetarian version, chop the meat into cubes and add to the wok and cook, making sure to seal the meat

- Add the onions, carrots and courgettes to the wok and cook for a few mins
- Add the 4-5 tablespoons of soy sauce to the wok and mix in, turning the heat down low to simmer for a few minutes
- Season with a pinch or two of salt and pepper
- Serve meal with rice brown rice when cooked

## **Vegan Rice Pudding – Serves 2 People (Delicious Hot or Cold)**

This dish works great either as a dessert – or as a breakfast, believe it or not!

1 cup of brown rice (½ cup per person)

2 tablespoons of desiccated coconut

¼ to ½ cup of goji berries

Up to ½ litre of either hemp, rice or coconut milk

## **Method**

- Boil 1 cup of brown rice in a saucepan of boiling water for 20-25 mins and then drain off

- Serve the rice in bowls with your choice of non-dairy milk

- Add desiccated coconut and goji berries to taste and mix them in

- Enjoy this lovely dish hot as a dessert

- To enjoy this as a quick and nutritious breakfast, simply add more milk and put the contents into a sealable container and put in the fridge.

- Enjoy this delicious dish the next morning for breakfast!

*Above recipe included with permission from Karen Lee of the Sensitive Foodie Kitchen* http://www.thesensitivefoodiekitchen.com

# CHAPTER SUMMARY

### Key Learning #1:
### Eating On Purpose is Crucial

The food you eat has a big impact on your health in general. Poor food choices will have a negative impact on your stress levels, energy levels, focus and concentration.

### Key Learning #2:
### Dispelling Food Myths

One of the biggest food myths ever is the lie that generations of people have been fed and that is that consuming dairy products will give you strong bones! Long term Consumption of Dairy products will actually do the opposite and lead to osteoporosis!

### Key Learning #3:
### Whole Food Plant Based is the Way Forward

Moving towards a whole food plant based diet is the way forward for optimum health. The good news is, you don't have to do it all at once, moving towards a plant based diet gradually over time is fine.

## *MY LEARNINGS & NEW COMMITMENTS*

_____

_____

_____

_____

_____

_____

_____

_____

_____

_____

_____

_____

_____

_____

_____

_____

_____

_____

_____

# Chapter 2:
# Get Your Thirst On

It is important to drink lots of water otherwise you will suffer from the effects of dehydration. So, what is dehydration? It's a condition caused by the excessive loss of water from your body; it causes a rise in blood sodium levels.

In this section we're going to cover three of the effects of dehydration:

- **Poor concentration**
- **Lethargy**
- **Weight gain**

Let's explore these 3 Effects of Dehydration in more detail below:

### Poor concentration

Your ability to concentrate becomes massively diminished when you are dehydrated. Did you know that 70% to 80% of the human body should be made up of water? Most people's body is not, because most people are in a chronic state of dehydration.

The brain is supposed to contain 83% water, so if you're even slightly dehydrated it's going to have a big impact on how your brain functions. Every cell in your body is made up of a high percentage of water, so dehydration will have systemic implications as well.

How does that relate to poor concentration? Well, being just 5% dehydrated can cause as much as a 25% decrease in your cognitive function – so water is clearly crucial. This prevents you from concentrating, you're not going to be able to focus as well as you would like and you are just not going to function as well as you could or should.

**Lethargy**

In addition, water is a huge source of energy for the body: not getting enough is going to cause fatigue and lethargy. As an essential nutrient for every cell in your body, water is extremely important for your comfort and well-being.

**Weight gain**

When you are dehydrated the cells of your body are depleted of energy. However, the body and the mind aren't good at distinguishing between being hungry and being thirsty; when you think you are hungry you are likely to be thirsty. But it gets worse: dehydration decreases your body's ability to burn fat and encourages excessive calorie consumption; it will also decrease your metabolism and that will lead to weight gain. So you can see how eating when you are actually thirsty can be extremely counter-productive to your general state of health and weight.

## REHYDRATION

We've now established that dehydration has a massive impact on your body and your body's ability to function well; rehydration will of course start to correct some of the above problems. Once you start to rehydrate yourself better, and maintain hydration, your body will function much better – and on a higher level.

My clients invariably ask how much water is 'enough'. As with so many aspects of health, it all depends: on your body size, your weight and your activity levels. You want to look to a minimum of two litres of water per day; although this figure is frequently encountered in the media, it is important to realise that this figure is only the baseline – the minimum. You want to look to two litres of water consumption *minimum* every day as opposed to it being the *optimum*.

Two to four litres per day is ideal; the more active you are, the more water you going to need to keep your body filled with the energy that water provides. Professional athletes can – and often need to – drink in excess of six litres of water per day.

## Best sources of water

Alkalised Ionized water from a water ionizer would be the ideal source of water for you to drink. Not only does an Alkalising Water ioniser take impurities out of the water, it also makes your water more alkaline and it ionises the water too. The water from a high quality alkalising water ioniser is so smooth and the quality and taste is far superior to water from any other source in my experience.

The second best option is a Reverse Osmosis system in your home. Reverse osmosis takes all of the impurities of the water which is great, the downside however is that it also removes some of the mineral content of the water as well.

The third best option there would be a jug filter system, such as those made by Brita, which are very inexpensive in comparison to the costs of a water ionizer or a reverse osmosis system. The place to start would depend on you budget of course. The gold standard really would be a water ionizer though, although that would require a bigger investment. Initially at the very least getting a filter jug would be far better than drinking tap water, so that all the water that you drink is going through a filter system.

## The worst sources of water

The worst source by far is to drink tap water. It's full of so many toxins, laden with heavy metals and drugs (that come from prescription drugs that people have consumed) and lots of bacteria. Essentially the water from a tap is rubbish; it's poor quality and depending on where you live, you can probably smell the chlorine in it as soon as you turn the tap on.

Another poor source of water is bottled water. Now, don't get me wrong, it's better than tap water because it's supposedly mineral water; however, some are better than others. Note, though, that this water is not necessarily particularly fresh: it's been lying in a warehouse in plastic bottles – which is a problem in itself, because some of the chemicals from the plastic bottle will leach into the water. In addition to that, those bottles of water have most likely been lying in a warehouse for months or even longer.

Another question clients often ask relates to the optimum time to drink. First thing in the morning is a great time to start your rehydration process: it will quench your thirst after six to eight hours of sleeping. You may like to have hot water in the morning: this will increase your metabolism more effectively – more so than drinking cold water or water at room temperature. You can also have a slice of lemon in there as well, to further increase the alkalisation process on your body.

In addition to this, drink regularly throughout the day; make sure you drink *before* you're thirsty – because when you feel thirst you are already significantly dehydrated. So, drink little and often and regularly, throughout the day. Don't wait until you are thirsty.

Stop drinking water about 30 minutes before you start to eat your meal and for about 30 minutes after you've eaten. This prevents dilution of the strong acids in the stomach, which are used to break up and metabolise the food that you eat.

## STRATEGIES FOR SUCCESS

In this section we are going to consider how best to:

- **Cultivate a drinking habit**
- **Invest in quality equipment**
- **Monitor your success**

### Cultivate a drinking habit

Like everything, it's very important to start with where you are at – and aim for slow and steady wins; slow and steady wins the race, as the saying goes. You can't go from zero all the way up to three to four litres of water per day in one fell swoop: that would be far too much of a jump, so you need to increase things gradually.

If you are not drinking any water at all right now, start off with a glass or two per day; slowly increase the volume that you are drinking each day over a few weeks until you eventually you get to the three to four litres of water per day – with two litres per day being your first big milestone.

An easy way to cultivate that drinking habit is to have a pint of water or glass bottle of water on your desk or in front of your workstation and by your bed. That way, if it's in a pint or similar size it's very easy to track. If you are having four pints of water a day then that is roughly two litres a day.

Another easy strategy to increase your water intake, if you are somebody who drinks tea and coffee regularly throughout the day, is to start to switch some of your teas and coffees for hot water instead.

## Invest in quality equipment

It's a large investment to get reverse osmosis fitted to filter all the water that comes into your house. However, although a big investment it will provide lots of very clean filtered water to drink – and also to bathe and shower in as well.

A more affordable piece of equipment that I would recommend you get is a water ionizer and that is much more affordable. The one I've got costs around £1,500 but you can usually pay for that over a period of time, typically one to two years. The make I've got is the Chanson Miracle Max Water Ionizer, but there are various different companies offering them – do an internet search to get more information.

If this sort of expenditure is too much of a stretch then, at the very least, get a Brita filter jug and start to filter the tap water that you may currently be drinking.

## Monitor your success

Get a tracking book to start to measure how much water you drink; as we've said before (and as the great Jim Rohn said before us!), "What's tracked and measured will improve".

Keeping a close eye on how much water you drink (or don't drink) is very powerful. I use a tiny notebook which you can take out, whenever and wherever, to document how much water you are drinking – and when. On each page I write the date, time and volume of water that I drink – when I drink it. Don't leave it until later, or you'll overlook it! Add it all up before bed, so you can monitor very easily how much you are drinking – and then you can track, measure and improve.

# CHAPTER SUMMARY

## Key Learning #1:
## Hydrate to Lose Weight

Dehydration is such a big factor in health and performance. Just 5% dehydration will decrease your cognitive function by up a huge 25%. Some of the direct or indirect effects of dehydration are lethargy, poor concentration and weight gain.

## Key Learning #2:
## Choose Water Sources Wisely

Rehydration (and maintaining that) will go a long way to correcting the symptoms of lethargy, poor concentration and weight gain.

We covered how much water is enough; the best sources of water; the worst sources of water and when is best to drink water. A minimum of two litres of water per day is needed; the gold standard in terms of equipment would be to have a water ionizer or reverse osmosis.

The worst sources of water would be tap water followed by bottled water. When to drink water? First thing in the morning is a great time to start your rehydration process and then little and often, throughout the day.

Importantly, drink *before* you are thirsty.

**Key Learning #3:**
**Track and Measure**

Get a thirst on. We talked about how to cultivate a drinking habit. Start at where you are at and gradually increase the amount of water that you drink each day. Slowly and steadily build up to three or four litres of water per day.

We talked about tracking and measuring how much water you are drinking; this will quickly improve your water intake.

## *MY LEARNINGS & NEW COMMITMENTS*

_____

_____

_____

_____

_____

_____

_____

_____

_____

_____

_____

_____

_____

_____

_____

_____

_____

_____

_____

# PART 2:
# MOVE ON PURPOSE

# Chapter 3:
# Improve Your Energy

Movement is an essential nutrient for your brain, it powers up the brain, so it's vital to move your body to cultivate energy.

## The Problems with Having a Lack of Energy

When you lack energy, it's more likely that you will use stimulants – to make you more alert and give you a boost. Stimulants might be coffee, energy drinks, cups of tea or lots of other sugary drinks that that give you a 'perceived boost'. The more that consumption of these stimulants increases, the more this leads to them becoming less and less effective.

These stimulants are highly addictive, when you first drank a coffee or energy drink years ago, it's highly likely that you got a high (big boost of energy) from it. Then over time your body down regulates (gets used to it) so you then need more and more of it to get the same effect and it keeps on down regulating so eventually you no longer get any effect from it at all!

I don't know whether you can relate to that? It is also very common for people who suffer from a lack of energy to go for high-sugar quick-fix snacks. That leads to insulin spikes and ultimately that leads to weight gain – and eventually diabetes, which is one of the leading causes of death in the western world today. That will increase the amount of acid in the body and this, in turn, is going to increase the stress response in the body as well, which we will cover later on in this book.

## MANAGING A LACK OF ENERGY

At the end of the day, nearly all of these problems arise because people do not focus on the triad of health: mindset, nutrition and exercise. Simply put, the problems of demotivation, poor energy and ultimately poor health result from this triad being out of balance.

That's where the Total Health Transformation programmes proven system comes into play, so before we consider what causes somebody to have poor motivation, energy and health, we have to go back to basics and ask ourselves what we mean by these words: 'motivation', 'energy' and 'health'. If we don't understand what they are, there's little chance of improving them! This is similar to a point made later in the book – if you can't assess something, you can't modify it.

- **Defining energy**

  This is the strength and vitality required for sustained physical and/or mental activity.

  Energy is life and life is energy, we are all made up of energy and we are all connected. People who speak with energy, passion and charisma can move you and inspire you to make a positive change in your life. It's because they have connected with you energetically on some level. Energy is enthusiasm and that is infectious! Enthusiasm and passion is what drives your energy levels, so it stands to reason that if you love what you do then you will have a high level of energy. Can you relate to that, how high is your energy?

## Move on purpose

Many people don't exercise at all and this is, literally, taking them into an early grave. Some people exercise a little, but many people don't exercise at all and that is a huge problem. Insufficient exercise is closely linked to coronary heart disease, increased cholesterol (the low-density lipoproteins (LDLs - the so-called 'bad cholesterol')).

Insufficient exercise also gives an increased risk of Alzheimer's disease, together with an increased risk of cancer; those who are inactive have been found to die much younger than those who are active. If you've been through periods of your life where you don't exercise much, you will have noticed that lack of exercise causes you to be lethargic. It massively affects your levels of motivation, it causes demotivation and ultimately contributes to poor health..

It's quite likely that you were aware that a lack of exercise is linked to heart disease. That's something that has been in the media for many years, and it's quite possible you are aware that lack of exercise has an impact on increasing your levels of cholesterol, the 'bad cholesterol' specifically. When you exercise, the so called 'good cholesterol', the high-density lipoproteins (HDLs) increase and the LDLs decrease. Conversely, if you don't exercise, HDLs (the good ones) decrease and LDLs (the bad ones) increase.

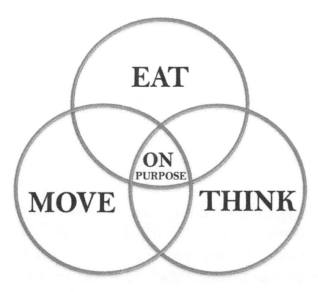

It's most likely, however, that you *weren't* aware that a lack of exercise increases your risk of Alzheimer's and dementia or your risk of cancer. So, exercise is *vital* to improve your motivation, your energy and, more importantly, your health.

## IMPLEMENTING *TOTAL HEALTH TRANSFORMATION EXERCISE*

I'm not going to stand here and say you need to go to the gym for three hours a day, every single day, seven days a week, 365 days of the year – although if you enjoy the gym, then do go regularly!

What I found over the years is that lots of people think they 'should' go to the gym or that they 'have to' go the gym. But once they get there, they hate being there. That is really counter-productive, so if you don't like going to the gym, then don't go! It may surprise you to hear that from me, but I'm all about *enjoying* what you do and doing what you love. If that doesn't include going to the gym for you then don't go.

Instead, find something that you love doing. That might be walking, going for a run, going swimming, walking the dog, dancing or indeed any activity you love to do! Whatever it is, as long as you're *moving* and you do it *regularly* it is good. Ideally, you should be exercising for at least one hour every day – but remember: the key is to enjoy it because you need to do it regularly for it to be effective. If you don't enjoy it, you're not going to do it regularly, it's as simple as that.

You may have joined a gym in the past and found yourself going for a few weeks at the beginning of the year when you're on a health kick. However, you possibly stopped going. I don't know whether you can relate to that? Gyms make so much money from people who subscribe to a membership – and then don't use it. Once again, find something that you love doing and do it regularly.

Two practices I have found to be very useful (and would certainly recommend) would be yoga and Pilates. I recommend Pilates to many of my coaching clients – and also to lots of my patients as a chiropractor. It's a very effective way of improving core stability and strengthening your core. If you ever had any physical problems, any spinal issues (like low back pain, or joint pain/injuries in general) Pilates is great for strengthening your body to prevent these injuries recurring. Yoga is fantastic for improving flexibility, and helps your body to move the way it's supposed to. I certainly recommend regular chiropractic check-ups as well, to keep your body moving well – and to ensure that your exercises are actually beneficial to your body.

How Do Your Current Exercise Habits stack up? Rate Your Current Fitness Score Below:

| Area | Out of 10 (10 Being Amazing!) |
|---|---|
| Strength | |
| Flexibility | |
| Energy & Vitality | |

## IMPROVE YOUR CURRENT FITNESS ROUTINE

### Not performing at your best? Symptoms of poor performance

To be truly healthy and be a peak performer, you need to eat, move, and think – on purpose. What do I mean by that? Eat on purpose, move on purpose, and think on purpose. Essentially that comes down to optimum nutrition, mastering your mind and moving your body – in other words, regular exercise. In this chapter, we're going to look at three symptoms of poor performance:

- **Poor appearance**
- **Poor stamina**
- **Lethargy**

#### Poor appearance

If you have a poor level of physical fitness, then that can lead to being overweight and being flabby – which can lead to lacking in confidence and negative internal self-talk. If you don't like the look of yourself, it's likely that you don't love yourself.

You can see that there's a strong link – and a lot of overlap – between the way you look and the way you talk to yourself. In other words, the way you feel. So, there is also a strong link between how you feel and how you look. A two-way street, if you like.

**Poor stamina**

If you're not moving your body, then you're not generating energy. That can lead to getting tired easily and not being able to see things through. Again, I'm sure you can see how this overlaps into other areas of life, because having adequate energy and stamina is a massive requirement for pretty much anything that you want to achieve.

**Lethargy**

Movement is an essential nutrient for the brain, as it powers the brain. Consider the analogy of a car: when you start a car, it starts because the battery provides enough energy to start; then you drive the car and the alternator comes into play and powers up the battery, which later provides the 'starting' energy.

Movement is the same sort of thing for us human beings; it is an essential nutrient for the brain. Much as the fuel that we put into our body, the food and the drink, are important for energy and thus to power the body, movement is an absolutely essential nutrient for your brain.

When we don't move our body, that can lead to tiredness, lethargy, exhaustion. Our body is designed to move regularly – it's not designed to be sedentary or to exercise very rarely, like so many people do today.

Did you know that sitting is as poor for your spine as sugar is for your teeth? I'm sure you'll agree that most people spend far too much time sitting down.

Take a moment to think how much time you spend sat down on your commute to work. Is it an hour to – and from – work? Maybe in your car or on the train or bus. Then, when you get to work, you probably sit in front of a computer for some – or most, or all – of the day. Then you get back on your commute back home.

When you do get home, you may sit on the couch, maybe watch a bit of TV and then have dinner at the dinner table. Maybe you eat your dinner in front of the TV, like so many people nowadays.

I'm sure you can see that we are, as a planet, basically sitting down way too much. It's not only causing damage to our spines. As we're talking about energy, it's also going to make you lethargic, have less stamina – and ultimately affect your physical appearance. Which puts you back into that vicious circle...

# TOTAL HEALTH TRANSFORMATION - CASE STUDY

My initial reason for getting involved in this programme was with the big goal of getting into the best shape of my life for my wedding.

At the beginning of the programme you helped me get a baseline for where I was starting from. Then I was able to track and measure everything going forwards with regards to my health, fitness routines, nutrition and daily mindset habits.

A revelation for me was learning how much water we should be drinking and how dehydrated I was to begin with! When I increased my water intake my energy levels skyrocketed and my clarity of thought improved exponentially as well!

Another big learning for me was to significantly cut down on my caffeine intake as I realised I had for many years been running on adrenaline fuelled by coffee! I used to definitely rely on caffeine, especially if I was going to be trading very late into the evenings. I've noticed there's no need for me to do that anymore just by getting all the right food combinations, the right food into my diet. Now I barely have any caffeine and my energy levels continue to increase every day.

I wanted to say a big thank you to Dr Danny! Since going through your Total Health Transformation programme I've achieved my goal of getting into amazing shape for my wedding day, which is fantastic! I've got great energy levels and I can only see that really increasing now as the months go on as I continue these positive habits and continue to learn more. It's a continual journey of constant and never ending improvement, you've really inspired me on that front and it's such a great place to be – thank you!

Phil Carr
Founder of The Gold & Silver Club

## What are the right exercises?

Different exercises suit different people. Even though you may be in a job that requires you to be moving around a lot, this is no substitute for a proper physical exercise programme.

So, what are the factors involved in the right exercises? That's a very personal choice; not only do different people *like* different things, they *respond to* and *need* different things. The four areas we're going to focus on in this section are:

- **Enjoyment**
- **Strength training**
- **Cardiovascular training**
- **Flexibility**

### Enjoyment

Lots of people go to the gym because they feel that they should rather than because they want to. These people end up quitting gym memberships very, very quickly. (And that ultimately makes the gym owners rich, so many people are paying for a service that they don't use!)

In January people tend to make new year's resolutions. They want to get fit – but, usually, before the end of January (and definitely before the end of February!) many have quit the gym, because they find they just don't enjoy it in the way they expected.

This is absolute madness, so simply find a form of exercise that you know you love doing. It will be far easier to stick doing this – walking, swimming, dancing or whatever it is – because it is something that you enjoy doing and you'll almost certainly find you stick to it.

A nice bonus of doing something regularly that you love doing is that you'll get a buzz from feeling you are able to do it – rather than the negative emotions of feeling persuaded or coerced into doing something. It's a completely different mindset, and what that does is to release lots of serotonin into your bloodstream and lots of endorphins. This gives a boost to all those different "feel-good" factors, which is obviously going to improve your health as well. All these hormones contribute to growth and repair in the body, which is what we want. The aim is to be constantly improving on a daily basis, whilst enjoying the process.

**Strength**
Strength training is important, as it keeps muscles healthy and bones strong. It makes you more able to handle what life throws at you. I must stress again that just because you might be in a physical job, that should not and does not

replace strength training. It's really important to do some resistance training (exercising your muscles) as well as simple cardio training (which exercises and strengthens your heart); they are both important, and so it's very important to do both.

Lifting weights or using your own body weight for exercises, is essential. This has lots of different benefits – it's going to increase muscle mass, speed up your metabolism and increase bone density, which will help to prevent osteoporosis (preventing brittle bones, where peoples break bones easily). It's also going to maintain and increase joint flexibility. There are many additional benefits to strength training – these are just a few!

**Cardiovascular training**

Cardio is very important and it contributes to having a healthy heart; when we exercise it's really important that we exercise to the point of breaking sweat. Why? Well, that's going to increase your heart rate, which increases your blood pressure as it pumps lots of blood around the body. This increases the transmission of oxygen round to all the different tissues and cells in the body.

It's also going to increase the rate at which you get rid of the toxins from your body; different muscles all contracting helps lymphatic drainage to help drain the body of toxins.

Here's a top tip for you: doing cardiovascular training work (for example running, cross training, cycling, or other cardio workouts) *after* strength training will help further with weight loss, if that is a goal of yours.

And here's another top tip. Cardio training alone speeds up your metabolism for around about two to three hours; whereas doing resistance work (ie some weights or weight exercises using your own body weight) is going to speed up your metabolism for 12 to 24 hours after exercise. So, it makes sense that a combination of these two is going to be fantastically beneficial for you and help you achieve your health goals.

### Flexibility

It is very important that you have flexibility both in life and your body. To have all strength and no flexibility is extremely bad. You often see that in bodybuilders, who may have really strong muscles – but they've got zero flexibility. Some of the big bodybuilders can barely put their arms behind their back or reach behind themselves.

Flexibility and strength are essential. But it's also extremely important to have balance. Everything that I teach is all about bringing balance back to the *body*, the *mind* and the *spirit*. So, with regards to flexibility it's crucial to develop and use a stretching programme. This is essential for 'spinal hygiene': all the different segments in your spine need to keep moving the way they were designed, so that your nervous system can do the job that it's supposed to —deliver the messages from the brain to the body and back again as efficiently as possible.

A couple of different types of exercise that you can do are Yoga and Pilates; they're both very good for flexibility and core stability. Yoga is generally better for the flexibility, and Pilates is generally better for core stability – although there's a crossover between the two.

## Strategies for success

So there are lots of different strategies for success with regards to your physical fitness; aspects of this that we should consider include:

- **Setting goals**
- **Designing your program**
- **Easing into it**
- **Reviewing your progress**

### Setting goals

It's crucial to set goals for your fitness – and for life in general. Setting goals gives you something to aim for and focuses your mind on achieving it. If you've got no plan, you're not going to achieve what you want to.

So, let's have a look at how to set a goal. We're going to use the **CREATE** acronym here, to give you an outline as to how create a goal the right way.

**C** is for concise and clear

**R** is for realistic. Make sure that that goal is realistic; stretch yourself, certainly, but make it is realistic to be able to achieve your goals and do your activities

**E** is for ecology. Is it safe for me and for others around me?

**A** is 'as if now'. In other words, make the goal as if in the present time – as if you've already achieved it, as you're achieving it now (see example below to make this clearer)

**T** is for time and towards positive. It's very important to put a time on the goal for achieving it

**E** is about the end step. How do you know that you've achieved it? Ie how do you know when to stop?

Let's give you an example of setting a goal the right way. Look at a goal for health, which might sound something like, "It is now ....(date) and I have just reached my ideal weight of …… (your desired weight) and I feel great and I look fantastic in my new suit." You simply identify the two variables needed.

Okay, so that is a really easy way of setting a goal that follows the acronym of "CREATE": being concise and clear, realistic, ecology, as if now, it's got a time frame on it and an end step.

**Designing your programme**

It's vital to start with where you are at. Everyone is at a different level, so a programme for someone who has never ever exercised before is going to be very, very different to somebody who's a regular marathon runner, for example. In my Total Health Transformation programmes, I design bespoke programmes for each of my clients, which are matched to the client's ability and health goals. In other words, where they are now is matched up with where they want to get to.

As well as starting from the 'here and now', it's necessary to build up gradually. Due to the compound effect, by taking small steps, one step at a time over a period of time, you will ultimately make massive achievements. Olympians look to increase their performance by one (or less than one) per cent at a time. Each seems insignificant – an extra two millimetres here, a hundredth of a second faster there – but over time the cumulative effect of those 'one per cents' adds up to a significant increase in performance.

## Easing into it

The key is steady improvement, session upon session, week upon week, month upon month, year upon year. Having a coach or a mentor makes it so much more achievable. The reason for that is because my role as a mentor is to hold you accountable; it's to celebrate successes – and it's also to help you to find solutions to problems.

Accountability is to do with making sure that my clients do what they say they're going to do and achieve what they intend to achieve. Celebrating success is something that most people don't do enough of – so it's important that when clients achieve successes along the way, we really make a big point of celebrating those successes.

Obviously, along the way there are going to be challenges, so we work through challenges and find solutions. We focus on solutions, not problems.

## Reviewing progress

The late great Jim Rohn, an American entrepreneur and motivational speaker, once said, "What gets tracked and measured, improves". So, it's crucial to track and measure your progress. That's done by reviewing things along the way. So, when I'm working with clients, I review things regularly, readjust if necessary and, where necessary, tweak different strategies along the way. This is the value of mentors, to provide that accountability.

The exercise aspect of programmes that I offer are very flexible and are tailored to the individual; as we've seen, different exercises work better for different people according to their health goals and their starting point.

# CHAPTER SUMMARY

### Key Learning #1:
### The symptoms of poor performance: poor appearance, poor stamina and lethargy

**Poor appearance**

To be truly healthy and perform at your best, you need to eat, move and think on purpose. Your appearance is going to be affected by how you move your body – and there can be massive overlap between how you feel and how you look.

**Poor stamina**

Poor stamina is going to be a big factor if you're not moving your body, so it's essential to find an exercise regime that works for you; stick to it and it will give you more stamina.

**Lethargy**

Lethargy is a big factor in poor performance. A big learning key was, *'sitting is for your spine what sugar is for your teeth'.* It's crucial to move the body, otherwise you become lethargic – and it will also cause damage to your body as well.

## Key Learning #2:
## The right exercises

The key learning's here were:

- Enjoyment for sustainability of exercise
- Strength training is crucial for health, strength and weight loss
- Cardio training is absolutely essential for heart health and more
- Flexibility is crucial for spinal and neurological hygiene.

## Key Learning #3:
## Strategies for success

- Setting goals the right way: tailored, bespoke, programmes are the way to go to achieve your goals
- Easing into it: it's very important to build up your exercise programme gradually; that way you stick to it.
- Review progress: what gets tracked and measured improves.

## *MY LEARNINGS & NEW COMMITMENTS*

_____

_____

_____

_____

_____

_____

_____

_____

_____

_____

_____

_____

_____

_____

_____

_____

_____

_____

# Chapter 4:
# Achieve Your Ideal Weight

Ultimately if you choose not to do what is outlined in the pillars above then the end result will be weight gain and all the associated health problems that accompany it.

## WHAT IS IDEAL?

A measure of your body, the body mass index (BMI) is a measure of the ideal weight. 'Normal' on the BMI scale is 18.5 to 25; 'overweight' is classed as between 25 and 30; readings in excess of 30 are termed 'obese'.

### How do you work out the BMI?

Basically, you take your weight (in kilograms) and divide it by your height (in metres); when you've got that figure, you then divide that answer by your height again: that will equal your BMI, your body mass index.

Here's the bad news. There are consequences to not being your ideal weight – or not even caring or trying to achieve it. In this section, we're going to discuss four of those potential consequences, and cover:

- **Obesity**
- **Anorexia**
- **Heart disease**
- **Diabetes**

## Obesity

In the western world, people are (generally) massively overfed and undernourished. The food that people consume usually has a high percentage of 'empty calorie dense food', which is also nutrient deficient. An awful lot of the food that people consume in the western world today is just full of empty calories. Far too many refined carbohydrates are consumed in the western diet; to a large extent, even the eastern world is becoming westernized in that respect.

There is an epidemic of obesity worldwide; sadly, the UK is right up there in the highest rankings alongside the USA. This obesity problem relates to, in large part, the foods that people consume; it is also to do with what's added to food and drink these days. So many different chemicals and preservatives and additives are added to food and drinks, which compound the worldwide obesity epidemic.

That's not to make an excuse for people being able to blame things on the food producers, but it's a fact: there is an awful lot of additives in food and drink these days. These additives just don't help people if they are trying to lose weight or even just trying to be healthy.

People don't tend to think long term; it's all about immediate gratification. If you have something from a fast-food outlet it's not going to make you fat or overweight immediately; people tend to think about their current needs (hunger) right now, and not to the medium-distant future. However, if you have a fast-food meal every day over the next three to six months, the compound effect is going to multiply over time. It's going to work against you and that happens insidiously – without you being aware of it. Eventually you'll be very overweight and very unhealthy, but that won't happen overnight, so we tend not to be aware of it – or aware of the causes.

## Anorexia

Generally speaking, the western world's problem is not under-eating; it's over-eating. I've mentioned anorexia in this section just to give the polar opposite to obesity; it is something that we have to be aware of, although by comparison it is quite rare.

Anorexia is an eating disorder: a mental health disorder or condition. It often develops out of anxiety about body shape and/or weight. Irrational and unhealthy fears develop – the sufferer is either excessively worried about being fat or has an overwhelming desire to be thin. We won't be focusing too much on this subject in this book as a large number of books have been written on this topic already.

## Heart disease

People for many years have assumed that heart disease is hereditary or genetic. As a practising chiropractor and also a Wellness Expert I have often heard patients or clients say, "Oh okay, heart disease, it's in the family, so I'm going to get it."

The reality is that heart disease is not, essentially, genetic and it's not hereditary. Yes, it can be common for family members to get the same diseases, but it's a disease of *lifestyle* not your *genes*. Just because your mum or dad had heart disease, for example, does not mean that you will get heart disease. However, if you eat, move and think in the same way as your parents then it's quite likely that you're going to get the same lifestyle diseases. The reality is that our genes have not changed over the last ten to twenty thousand years; what has changed, however, is our environment, which has changed dramatically.

There is another myth around heart disease, which has been spread for the past three decades or more, and that is the cholesterol myth. Cholesterol is not the bad guy, and neither is fat. The bad guy which is causing people to be overweight and missing their ideal weight is sugar! High cholesterol has never ever been shown scientifically to cause heart disease. The story that high cholesterol *causes* heart disease is a complete myth, as it is simply not true; there are plenty of books on that subject, and I'd suggest that you look at a few of them, starting with *The Cholesterol Myth.*

## Diabetes

Type 2 diabetes is reaching record levels worldwide; sadly, there are more and more children getting diabetes and this is because they are eating, moving and thinking deficiently. In other words, they are not eating, moving and thinking on purpose the way they really need to if they / their parents want to be healthy.

There is so much sugar in so many of the different foods that most people eat most of the time; that food group is primarily refined carbohydrates. As a general rule, I would say all the different white pastas, white sugars, white rice, white bread and biscuits and crisps etc. – all of these are heavily refined and full of poor quality ingredients. I would go as far as to say, **"White is shite,"** because most of these refined carbohydrates are so sugar-laden that they put your body on a blood sugar rollercoaster.

Eating some of the food – whether it be a piece of bread or a cake or whatever – causes a big spike in your blood sugar; these foods, the refined carbohydrates, are very high on the glycaemic index, which is a measure of how quickly sugar can be released into your body. By eating lots of these different refined carbohydrates straight after you come down from this big sugar spike, you're going to be craving more foods that are also high on the glycaemic index. So, it's a vicious cycle: refined carbohydrates cause you to eat more of them: and that all contributes to, and is a big cause of, type 2 diabetes.

## KNOW WHAT'S RIGHT FOR YOU: IT'S NOT WHAT YOU THINK!

To know what's right for you, you need to look at the big picture; you need to consider all three of the following:

- **Eat on purpose (nutrition)**
- **Move on purpose (exercise)**
- **Think on purpose (mindset)**

These all play a vital role in achieving and maintaining your ideal weight, so we will now have a look at mindset, nutrition and exercise – and what you need to do in each of those areas of your life.

### Nutrition

All calories are not created equal. For the past two or three decades there has been an obsession with counting calories. Different foods contain different amounts of calories but these calories are not created equally. In recent times people have been mistakenly looking to a low-fat diet in order to lose weight and they've struggled as a result. People have been persuaded that fat is the enemy.

The reality is generally that low fat equals high sugar. There is a whole industry based around the idea that fat is the enemy and that fat makes people put on weight. Low fat is king, you are persuaded each day in the newspapers and TV programmes or advertisements. In reality, that is not the case.

However, if you take out the fat you need to replace it with something to give it an appealing taste. What do manufacturers do? They put significant quantities of sugar in these low-fat foods, so although they can be correctly described as low fat, they do not make you lose weight. In fact, quite the opposite! Just by being aware of this enables you to make very simple changes in order to be able to achieve and maintain your ideal weight.

## Exercise

Exercise is a crucial part of being able to achieve and maintain your ideal weight. The reality is that most people are lazy; this problem is compounded by not having enough energy to exercise, because people are eating the wrong foods – empty calories with no or very poor nutrition. We need to exercise for good health, but an added bonus is that you will feel good and you will look good as a result.

People need to realise that exercise is an essential part of health – it is not just something undertaken to look good. It's not about getting a beach body and having big muscles when you're on holidays and whatnot. It is about eating, moving and thinking to be healthy – i.e. on Purpose.

## Mindset

Stress levels play a big factor in whether you do or do not achieve (or maintain) your ideal weight. Remember that an increase in stress results in a constant stress response in your body – and that leads to an increase in cortisol, an increase in adrenaline released into your body, and that in turn leads to craving of sugar and fats to replace the energy supplies. Even if you are sitting at your desk, in front of your computer, your body cannot distinguish whether you're running from a lion or sitting still. All it knows is that stress hormones are being released into the body, so the stress response occurs.

When that stress response occurs when you're in work, you're not in a position to be able to go and burn off all of the energy that's just been released into the blood stream. All of those chemicals (cortisol and adrenaline) mean that you're going to crave sugar and fat; and that is going to make it really, really difficult for you to be able to achieve and maintain your ideal weight. The key is to eat, move, and think on purpose – ie do things deliberately, when you plan, rather than when your body is simply giving you the urge to do them.

## TIPPING THE SCALES IN THE RIGHT DIRECTION

So, as we look to tip the scales in the right direction going forwards, we'll focus on four key areas:

- **Setting goals**
- **Designing your programme**
- **Easing into it**
- **Reviewing progress**

### Setting goals

If you have already looked at Chapter 3 you will have encountered this, but a recap is always worthwhile. You need to set small goals initially so they can be quite easily achieved – and then you can build on that achievement and stretch yourself with bigger goals as you move forwards.

We're going to use the **CREATE** acronym here, to give you an outline as to how create a goal the right way.

> **C** is for **concise** and **clear**
>
> **R** is for **realistic.** Make sure that that goal is realistic; stretch yourself, certainly, but make it is realistic to achieve your goals and do your activities

**E** is for **ecology.** Is it safe for me and for others around me

**A** is '**as if now**'. In other words, make the goal as if in the present time – as if you've already achieved it, as you're achieving it now (see example below to make this clearer)

**T** is for **time** and **towards positive**. It's very important to put a time on the goal for achieving it

**E** is about the **end step. H**ow do you know that you've achieved it? Ie how do you know when to stop?

Let's give you an example of setting a goal the right way. Look at a goal for health, which might sound something like, "It is now ....(date) and I have just reached my ideal weight of ...... (your desired weight) and I feel great and I look fantastic in my new suit." You simply identify the two variables needed.

Okay, so that is a really easy way of setting a goal that follows the acronym of 'CREATE': being concise and clear, realistic, ecology, as if now, it's got a time frame on it and an end step.

### Designing your programme

When you're trying to make any change in your life (in this instance we're talking about achieving your ideal weight) it's important you should focus on adding in some positive habits or some positive foods, rather than depriving yourself of foods that you know you shouldn't be eating. For example, if you wanted to stop eating chocolate over a period of time, I'd always recommend focussing on starting to add some 'good' foods before, or at least alongside, stopping the 'bad' foods. Maybe add an apple to your diet each day. Then, over time, you can add in more and more good foods, more positive habits, more positive healthy foods. Eventually you'll add in so many good, healthy foods that you will no longer crave what you could call the 'bad' foods or the unhealthy food that all of us crave from time to time.

The reason for this is to avoid deprivation. When you deprive yourself of some food or drink, that's going to create or turn on a stress response in your body; that leads to an increase in cravings of sugar and fat. What do you reach for then? Refined carbohydrates … and the cycle continues.

So, we focus on *adding*, we do not *deprive*; that would be a recipe for disaster. We take things one step at a time, we set small achievable goals and we start with where we are at. We are not all at the same level, so start with where you are at right now.

## Easing into it

Consistent daily action, day on day, week on week, is where all the magic happens. It's very important that you ease into something like this gradually. One way that this is really effective is by being part of a 'group' – which can be as small as two people, or as large as a large class. Being part of a coaching group or a mentoring group holds you accountable for your actions; that accountability is the biggest reason for success in their lives.

In the coaching and mentoring groups that I run in the **Total Health Transformation** programmes, my clients tell me that this accountability is the single biggest and most powerful factor in their success.

## Reviewing your progress

"What is tracked and measured, improves," is a famous quote from the late great American entrepreneur Jim Rohn. Regular reviews with my private clients ensure they succeed in achieving their goals – whatever they are. It is essential to set these goals, measure them – and sometimes readjust them along the way where necessary.

If you need to change direction, if you need to change a habit, then you are allowed to do so. The process of change is different for every person; it's not like a cookie cutter, where everybody gets the same prescription to make the changes in their lives. Everybody has got a different situation, everybody is at a different stage in their life and, most likely, a different stage in their health journey too.

Any good coach or mentor will always ensure that health or fitness programmes are bespoke, and specific to the individual client. I run 1-to-1 programmes as well as group coaching, but even within a group I always ensure that the detail of the programme is specific to the individual client.

# TOTAL HEALTH TRANSFORMATION - CASE STUDY

"Just under 6 months ago, life was more than a bit of a struggle! I had great difficulty in standing up from a chair, walking up stairs and riding my bike was just out of the question! It was impossible for me to do any physical tasks and our other hobby of ballroom dancing was being severely hampered! I had a lot of pain especially in my knees and I generally felt very run down and tired most of the time!

Now six months later – **WOW what a change!**

We've just come back from our holiday where we went on several bike rides, one being over 5 miles and the other one just less than 20 miles! Incredible! Thank you, Dr. Danny! My wife and I also went for walks along the beach, the longest being a 6-mile walk – something I could have only dreamed about 6 months ago!

Your Coaching Programme was very easy to follow and thanks to your very simple diet recommendations I've now lost over 3 stone in the last 3 months which is amazing! I've now got more energy than I've had in the last 25 years which is great because we have a very active retirement planned! I just wish I'd known about your programme sooner Danny!"

**John Fisher – Retired Business Man**

# CHAPTER SUMMARY

## Key Learning #1:
## Consequences of not achieving your ideal weight

Some of these are:

- **Obesity**
- **Coronary heart disease**
- **Diabetes**

All of these are *lifestyle* diseases and they are completely preventable – and, in lots of cases, reversible.

## Key Learning #2:
## The big picture needs to be considered

Deficiencies and how people eat, move, and think all contribute to weight problems. Mindset stress is a big contributor in not achieving your ideal weight. People have been misled for decades: it's not *fat* that is the issue if you're trying to lose weight, the big issue really is *sugar*.

People are inherently lazy and this is compounded by poor nutritional choices; this makes a lot of people struggle to achieve – and maintain – their ideal weight.

## Key Learning #3:
## Do things - *on purpose*

If you want to get – and remain – healthy, you need to eat, move, and think on purpose. If you want to make permanent changes, and achieve and keep your ideal weight, then you need to make eating, moving and thinking on purpose a habit that becomes hard-wired within you. Make positive exercise, nutrition and mindset a lifestyle choice and a necessity. It's a 'must do', never mind, "Oh, I'll go on a diet for a bit". If you want to get healthy and stay healthy then you need to eat, move and think well *consistently*.

It's absolutely essential to set goals – and then be held accountable to make sure that you achieve them. Track and measure, and adjust course if required; really focus on adding positive healthy habits and different food groups and drinks. Do that one step at a time: one foot forward in front of the other, and you'll get to where you want to get to.

## *MY LEARNINGS & NEW COMMITMENTS*

_____

_____

_____

_____

_____

_____

_____

_____

_____

_____

_____

_____

_____

_____

_____

_____

_____

# PART 3: THINK ON PURPOSE

# Chapter 5:
# Improve Your Mindset

Your mindset is the key to success in all areas of your life, lets dive deep into the subject in this chapter.

## PROBLEMS OF POOR MINDSET

It's essential to start your day with the right mindset, *before* meditation. Set intentions for the day and practise gratitude. These are both ways of instructing the universe as to what you want to happen in your day; that way *you* can then be in charge of what happens in your day, rather than being at the mercy of other people's plans. Once you've set your day off in the right way, you'll be ready to go into your meditation in the right frame of mind.

When people are demotivated, lots of different things can happen. They may struggle to get out of bed, suffer from depression and often feel as if people are looking down on them. These people are generally not clear on their values and their life purpose; this exacerbates the problem and demotivates them further. This has a massive effect on their choices with regards to their nutrition, mindset and exercise – and is very detrimental to these three areas.

They are not able to eat well, move well or think well – and, again, they become increasingly demotivated as a result. They lack drive and determination; the demotivated person or business owner is more likely to use stimulants and alcohol in order to give them a pick-me-up or try to escape from their problems. It's not going to happen in all cases, but it does seem to be more and more common.

## MANAGING DEMOTIVATION

At the end of the day, nearly all of these problems arise because people do not focus on the triad of health: mindset, nutrition and exercise. Simply put, the problems of demotivation, poor energy and ultimately poor health result from this triad being out of balance.

That's where the Total Health Transformation programmes proven system comes into play, so before we consider what causes somebody to have poor motivation, energy and health, we have to go back to basics and ask ourselves what we mean by these words: 'motivation', 'energy' and 'health'. If we don't understand what they are, there's little chance of improving them! This is similar to a point made later in the book – if you can't assess something, you can't modify it.

- **Defining motivation**

  Motivation is defined as a process that initiates, guides and maintains goal-oriented behaviours. Motivation is what causes us to act, whether it's getting a glass of water to reduce thirst or reading a book to gain knowledge. It involves biological, emotional, social and cognitive forces that activate behaviour In your life and in business, motivation is that spark that gets you out of bed in the morning, that excitement that drives you towards your goals, that energy and perseverance to keep on track even when the going gets tough. With the right motivation and drive there is nothing that's out of reach for you, you can do it!

# THINK ON PURPOSE

All success begins with having the right approach. A positive mindset is absolutely essential – when your head is the right place, the rest just falls into place and becomes so much easier. An improved mindset strengthens your motivation, it boosts your energy and gives you an improved positive outlook; it has a huge positive impact on your health too. It's been scientifically proven that negative thoughts are ten times more powerful than positive ones; in simple terms, you need to have ten positive thoughts to neutralise just one negative thought. Now, this has massive connotations if you break it down and think about it.

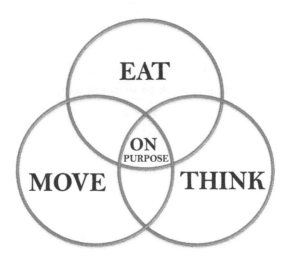

## How to implement a positive mindset

It's an ongoing constant process or cycle to maintain a positive mindset. It's not a simple journey: you don't get there and become enlightened. It's an ongoing journey that requires persistence. It requires eating, moving and thinking on purpose most of, if not all of the time.

The gratitude list that we talked about briefly (when you get up in the morning write a list of the ten things that you're grateful for) can be supercharged for even greater success. For each of those things you are grateful for, write down *how it makes you feel*.

That really supercharges the power of the gratitude, so take a moment out to start off a gratitude journal and then write a few sentences, a short paragraph, to set out your intention for the day. It's very powerful indeed to have a plan because if you *"fail to plan you plan to fail"*, to quote Benjamin Franklin.

The next thing to do after setting your intention is to meditate for 20 minutes as instructed in the next chapter. I would strongly recommend going on a permanent media diet: minimise and eventually eliminate watching the news, reading the newspapers and such like, as that will enable you to have a positive mindset far more easily.

Another good technique to practise regularly is **Emotional Freedom Technique** (EFT) which has often been nicknamed acupuncture without the needles! It's fairly new, and there are a lot of different teachers out there, so do an internet search and find out more about the subject; there's likely an EFT practitioner near you.

How Do Your Current Mindset Habits stack up? Rate Your Current Emotional Health Score Below:

| Area | Out of 10 (10 Being Amazing!) |
|---|---|
| Clarity of Thought | |
| Ability to Relax | |
| Quality & Quantity of Sleep | |

## IMPLEMENTING *TOTAL HEALTH TRANSFORMATION MINDSET*

There are many different things you can do to improve your mindset, some of which we will be covering in much more detail later. Let's just gently introduce some now, so you don't immediately get overwhelmed! A very good daily practice, ideally first thing in the morning, is to write a 'gratitude list' or to keep a 'gratitude journal'. I list ten things that I'm grateful for – and next to each item on that list, I indicate how it makes me feel to be grateful for that particular thing.

I'll give you an example. I note my thanks for my family; how does that make me feel? Well, it makes me feel loved and supported. Similarly, 'thank you for my mentors.' How does that make me feel? That makes me feel guided and supported. 'Thank you for my health.' How does that make me feel? That makes me feel blessed and really happy. 'Thank you for my friends.' How does that make me feel? Loved and supported.

I'm sure you can gather how that could apply to yourself. There are lots of different things that we all can be grateful for, things that we usually take for granted. It doesn't matter if they are small or big; there are lots and lots of things to be grateful for and acknowledging them puts us in a positive, powerful mindset for the day. So, that's the gratitude list.

Another key part of this morning ritual is setting your intention for the day. This is unbelievably powerful and I consistently reap the rewards of setting my intention for the day – every day. When we don't do this, we go about our day without anything specific to achieve, wondering aimlessly. However, when we set out our intentions and plans then we can map out how we want to feel for the day, and just what we want to achieve for the day. A theme we introduce later is that of being able to measure things; this also applies to our plans for the day. If we don't know what we intended to do in any one day, how will we know if we achieved them?

An example could be:

**_I intend to say yes to life and focus on the positive outcomes for myself, my friends, and my family. I intend to do meditation two times today and feel the peace of mind that brings me. I intend to exercise today and to really enjoy the process and feel really good and energised._**

There are lots of different things that you can do to set your intention on for each day, and it really helps focus your conscious and subconscious mind on achieving that intention for the day. I can't overstate how powerful this very simple strategy is. Give it a go – now! Take a moment out and jot down three or four things you would like to accomplish today or tomorrow. Then, at the end of the day, check to see how close you got to achieving them.

I urge you to have a go at that and really put some effort into it and really enjoy it. Watch what happens in your life when you are grateful and when you set out your positive intention for the day. I reckon you will really see your life transform over the next few weeks and months.

At the other end of the process is a truly powerful act to do before you go to bed: make a list of at least five things that have been successful for you that day. That could be something big – or something small. You might have had a success by getting some new clients into your business, or had a really successful day eating healthy foods, or maybe you went to the gym and had a really great workout session, or meditated that day or went for a nice peaceful walk. All of these events are your 'successes', and it is really empowering to note, acknowledge and celebrate them.

It is essential to give yourself a pat on the back when you are successful: every little helps to build and maintain momentum!

Here are a few powerful strategies that you can implement right away, to set up your day with the correct mindset from the second you get up in the morning. In the coming chapters I will be sharing lots more tips and strategies so you can implement the *Total Health Transformation* mindset into your day on a consistent basis. I will be sharing how to meditate effectively, and show how Emotional Freedom Technique (EFT) has had such a positive effect on my clients' businesses and their lives.

# CHAPTER SUMMARY

### Key Learning # 1:
### How to Avoid Overwhelm

Most people tend to focus far too much on doing the wrong things; this stems from having a lack of clarity, a scatter-brain approach to life, negative self-talk and being overwhelmed.

### Key Learning # 2:
### Media Free Diet

Eating, moving and thinking on purpose will enable you to have or develop the ability to focus on doing the right things. Be sure to eat well, keep blood sugar levels steady and be sure to exercise regularly: you'll be able to relax better for your meditation and focus on reducing exposure to the media – or, even better, go on a media-free diet.

### Key Learning # 3:
### Let it Go – Twice a Day

Negative thoughts are never going to go away. It's not a case of getting rid of them, but rather a case of changing your relationship with negative thoughts. Put yourself in a position of power, rather than in a position of weakness.

Meditation in the morning will allow your body to release the stresses that have accumulated in your subconscious and conscious mind whilst sleeping; meditation in the evening releases the stresses that have accumulated in the daytime. Meditation allows you to clear a lot of stress out of your body and your mind.

## *MY LEARNINGS & NEW COMMITMENTS*

_____

_____

_____

_____

_____

_____

_____

_____

_____

_____

_____

_____

_____

_____

_____

_____

_____

_____

# Chapter 6:
# Embrace the Power
# of Meditation

Meditation has been around for thousands of years and yet it is only today that its starting to become more mainstream in the western world.

## Focusing on the Wrong Things

Most people tend to focus on the wrong things, and in this section we'll focus on four specific issues:

- **Lack of clarity**
- **A scatter-brained approach to life**
- **Negative self-talk**
- **Being overwhelmed**

Meditation will help to rectify all of these issues.

## Lack of clarity

Having no clear plan for the day inevitably leads to getting very little done. Without setting clear objectives or making a plan for your day, you risk becoming part of somebody else's plans! Having a lack of clarity leads to frustration, anxiety and – of course – going round in a circle, which in turn perpetuates those feelings of frustration and anxiety.

## Scatter-brained approach to life

So many people are trying to do everything: they've got too much on their plate. They are trying to do a little bit of everything and becoming a jack-of-all-trades – but a master of none, which leads to achieving very little.

There are so many distractions these days, with so many different technologies and social media; this has a massive effective on your ability to focus. With so many distractions it's extremely easy to get distracted and off the point.

Trying to do everything can mean that you often find it very difficult to relax and switch off; inevitably, that makes you feel that you haven't got time to relax – so you don't make time for it.

## Negative self-talk

It's really important to recognise that very few of us will ever truly get rid of negative self-talk, so it's a case of changing your relationship with it. It's important to accept that, as you grow and evolve, fears are bound to come up; fears inevitably lead to more negative self-talk.

It's a case of learning to handle that and learning to feel the fear and do it anyway. That's actually the title of a fantastic book I read about 25 years ago. I've still got a copy on my bookshelf and I would definitely recommend it today: *"Feel The Fear And Do It Anyway"* by Susan Jeffers.

So, rather than focusing on stopping negative self-talk, focus on adding positive habits and positive thoughts into your life and your daily routines. The simple rationale is that you can crowd out the negative self-chatter with positivity.

## Being overwhelmed

When you take on too many projects it's easy to get overwhelmed. It's crucial that, in both your home and in your business life that, you learn to say no. Most people don't say no anywhere near enough; it comes back, again, to not having a plan, not having a vision and not setting your intention for the short, medium and long term. Inevitably, therefore, this is going to lead to being overwhelmed.

## GETTING A GRIP

In this section, we are going to consider:

- **How to meditate**
- **When to meditate**
- **How to support meditation**
- **How to implement a positive mindset**

All of these things will teach you how to get a grip in your life.

### How to meditate

There are lots of different styles of meditation; the style of meditation I've been doing for many years is known as **transcendental meditation** (TM), which is a technique for promoting a state of relaxed awareness. I'm not a TM teacher, so if you'd like to know more about the topic go on to the internet and search for 'transcendental meditation. Learn more about it and find a local TM centre where a trained and qualified TM teacher will be able to teach you. I would strongly recommend learning TM, as it's been a game changer for me! There are hundreds of research papers proving its efficacy, and it is the most research-backed type of meditation that you can do.

### When to meditate

I would recommend meditating twice a day, for 15 to 20 minutes each time. I find is a great time to

In this section, though, we will concentrate on **mindfulness meditation:** basically, focusing on your breathing. When you do this sit comfortably in a chair, with your feet flat on the floor; rest your hands on your lap and close your eyes.

Begin to focus on your body, beginning to imagine the air entering your mouth going into your lungs, oxygenating the body and then breathing the air back out again. Really slow down and focus on the breathing as if there is nothing else to focus on, just the breathing.

Don't worry if any thoughts pop into your head; they will do, so just acknowledge those thoughts, thank them and then let them go – and just return to focusing on the breathing. It will take some practice to get used to this, like most things in life though! Practice makes perfect, so it will get easier and more natural over time.

meditate is first thing in the morning; the second meditation I'd recommend either before your dinner or as the last thing at night, before bed.

## How to support meditation

Make sure you're well hydrated: drink plenty of water, as that will definitely aid your ability to relax and get more out of your meditation. Minimise or eliminate the consumption of stimulants: definitely do not drink teas and coffees or alcohol before, during or after meditation. Make sure you eat very well: focus on optimum nutrition, get plenty of sleep and also go on a media-free diet – no computers, tablets, television or newspapers! This is especially true first thing in the morning and last thing at night.

People who read newspapers and watch the news religiously first thing in the morning (and last thing at night) will start (and end) the day by activating a stress response; this does nothing to help cultivate a positive mindset. Let's face it, nearly everything in the news is to do with negativity and is fear-based, so that starts a stress response in your body. Starting and ending the day with that is definitely not going to be good for your health!

# CHAPTER SUMMARY

### Key Learning #1:

Get Clarity in your life and be sure to focus on one thing at a time otherwise you will suffer from overwhelm. Have a clear plan for what you want to achieve in the day

### Key Learning #2:

Make time to relax and switch off, especially when you think you "haven't got time to relax!" That's where meditation comes in to its own.

### Key Learning #3:

Pick a style of Meditation that resonates with you, whether that be TM, Mindfulness, Guided Meditation. Whatever style you choose, do it often and you will reap the benefits

# *MY LEARNINGS & NEW COMMITMENTS*

_____

_____

_____

_____

_____

_____

_____

_____

_____

_____

_____

_____

_____

_____

_____

_____

_____

_____

# Chapter 7:
# Relax and Sleep
# Like a Baby

Sleep is so important both in terms of optimal health and peak performance. Let's explore the causes and consequences of not getting enough sleep.

## CAUSES OF EXHAUSTION

There are countless reasons for exhaustion; in this chapter, we're going to focus on just four in the context of peak performance and health:

- **Insomnia**
- **Anxiety**
- **Irrational fears**
- **Lack of time off**

### Insomnia

This is pretty obvious – not enough sleep is going to lead to being exhausted. As a result of that, poor concentration is going to occur. And then, if you're not concentrating well, you're clearly going to make more errors in whatever you're doing. Insomnia is a massive stressor to your adrenal glands: essentially, you'll be 'running on adrenaline', a phrase I'm sure you've heard before. This brings a risk of adrenal exhaustion – and, because you are exhausted, this likely increases the use of stimulants, coffees and teas and energy drinks. Stuff like that simply causes more and more adrenal stress and this exacerbates the stress response. Then you've got a classic vicious circle that you will find increasingly hard to break out of.

## Anxiety

This is very closely linked to poor sleep quality. It links into repeatedly firing the adrenals, always running on adrenaline; lots and lots of stress hormones are constantly being pumped into the blood. Consequently, somebody who is anxious is said to be quite often *always on edge* and they find it difficult to relax. This cycle also tends to perpetuate itself and it's very, very draining – as you possibly already know...

## Irrational fears

When you're not sleeping very well, you're constantly anxious. The stress response is constantly in action in your body. This is because the stress hormones are constantly being pumped around your body, your brain and your bloodstream; this leads to many, many different things that cause havoc with your ability to relax. Two of the main stress hormones involved in the stress response are Cortisol and noradrenalin.

So, all of these stress hormones constantly circulating in your body cause you to become overly sensitive and increasingly fearful; this in turn leads to increasing anxiety. It's going to decrease your short-term memory, it's going to decrease your ability to concentrate, it's going to decrease serotonin levels in your body – which is going to affect your ability to relax and sleep and to feel good. So, all of these different factors relate to the stress response that happens in your body.

## Lack of time off

The last thing that causes exhaustion (well, the last thing that we're going to talk about in this chapter, anyway) is a lack of time off, a lack of rest. Each of the previous three items is exacerbated by overwork – and this whole thing is a vicious cycle. All of the above contribute to exhaustion – but they also contribute to each other, thus compounding that vicious circle.

# RELAXATION

Relaxation is really important; it allows the body time to regenerate. A lot of growth and repair happens when we're sleeping – when we make time to relax, this ultimately increases our energy and increases our productivity. Different components of relaxation come from the same three areas:

- **Mindset –** *Thinking on Purpose*
- **Nutrition –** *Eating on Purpose*
- **Exercise –** *Moving on Purpose*

## Mindset

Being relaxed allows for a positive mindset to come to you much more easily; it's an awful lot easier to maintain, as well. By getting adequate rest that leads to increased productivity, increased energy, increased motivation and ultimately increased health.

There is a term known as ***"the golden four"*** – the time between 10pm and 2am (when most of the physical regeneration in your body happens) and again between 2am and 6am (when more of the psychological, emotional repair and regeneration happens). Getting plenty of sleep is **essential** to a healthy state of mind.

It's been proven scientifically over the past couple of decades that a positive outlook is absolutely essential for your health; it's also a proven fact that when you're around somebody or something negative, that's going to have a negative impact on your health. We can say, simplistically, "what you think about you bring about" – so if you're constantly stressed out, anxious, angry, then you're going to attract even more of those stressed-out, anxious and angry things and thoughts.

## Nutrition

What you eat (or don't eat) and what you drink (or don't drink) has a huge impact on your ability to relax. Did you know, for example, that if you're just **5%** dehydrated that's going to reduce your cognitive ability by up to 25%? Water is very important, because most of our body should be water. Most people have no idea what percentage of the body should be water; it's a surprise to find out that our body is between 70 and 80% water, and the brain contains even more – around 83%. So, is it any wonder that dehydration is a massive factor in your ability to have energy and, ultimately, your ability to relax at the end of the day.

Some foods will aid your ability to relax and aid rejuvenation growth and repair; others, on the other hand, will do the opposite and cause anxiety, exhaustion, and cell damage. So, it's hardly rocket science to say that you should know which foods and drinks bring about which outcome, so you can make better health decisions based on optimum nutrition.

## Exercise

Movement is an absolutely essential nutrient for the brain; it powers the brain up. An analogy I always use as a chiropractor when running health workshops is to compare the body to a car. As you start and then drive a car, the alternator charges the battery. In a human being, movement of the human body charges up the brain, charges up the body and gives us energy. Of course, we need to get energy from food and drink, but movement is an absolutely essential nutrient for your brain: I term this 'movement nutrition'.

Exercise releases endorphins, dopamine and serotonin into your bloodstream and your body; these all make you feel good and they allow the body to relax more easily. When you exercise, this aids the release of toxins from the body and encourages an increase of oxygen around the body. In turn there is also an increase in oxygen to the brain and this helps you focus and relax better – and ultimately you'll be able to be more relaxed and be calmer.

## HOW TO SLEEP LIKE A BABY!

These same three components (mindset, nutrition and exercise) help you sleep like a baby. At the end of this section, we will put it all together and go through some techniques that you can implement yourself to be able to begin to sleep like a baby – tonight!

### Mindset

There are loads of different techniques with regards to mindset to be able to relax better and then sleep better. There's meditation, emotional freedom technique

(EFT). The 'Total Health Transformation Stress Buster' is a technique that I like to use a lot – and then there are positive daily rituals as well, such as 'daily gratitude' (setting an intention for the day first thing in the morning) which really set up your day for success!

I find it very useful to severely limit the amount of media to which I expose myself: I avoid reading newspapers and I avoid watching the news. That allows me to be a lot more chilled, because reading the newspapers and watching the news really stresses people out; in my opinion, the worst thing you can do is watch the news as soon as you get up in the morning and/or watch the news last thing before bed. It's going to stress you out and you're not going to be able to sleep well, so my advice is to follow my example: avoid newspapers and avoid watching the news. I introduced this in Chapter 5, but here it is again.

## Daily gratitude

I like to practise 'gratitude' in the morning and in the evening; it's a really simple exercise. When you get up, take a journal (or start a journal if you don't do that already); put the date at the top and then write down 10 things that you're grateful for right now. If you want to supercharge this philosophy though, put down a reason why you're grateful for each item / thing as well. In other words, what are you grateful for and why?

An example of that might be:

*"Thank you for my family." **How does that make me feel?** "I feel love and support or loved and supported."*

Other examples could be:

*"Thank you for my healing." **How does that make me feel?** "That makes me happy."*

*"Thank you for a great day at work. **How does that make me feel?** "I feel joy from that,"*

Finally, I also write a very short paragraph (no more than four or five lines) to set my intention for the day. It's very important to outline how you want your day to be so you can attract lots of good things into your day.

*Positive Intentions*

Set an intention for the day. I will give you an example: I am a Chiropractor and Peak Performance Consultant, so an intention might be:

**"I intend to have 5 new patients today at Crawley Chiropractic Centre; I intend to have fun in all that I do today. I intend to help several new Coaching clients today begin their journey back to health! I intend to say yes to life and focus on success, love, peace, happiness – and focus on having fun, thank you, thank you, thank you."**

That's just an example of an intention that I wrote a few days ago; when you set your intention first thing in the morning (or, even better, the night before, just as you're going to bed) you plan to have a day that *you* want, rather than sitting back and having things happen to you.

These are just simple exercises on improving your mindset and helping you to relax better; there are many other techniques that can be adopted, and most of these will be covered in later chapters.

## Nutrition

Lots of different foods enhance your ability to relax – and therefore enhance your ability to be able to sleep. Any food that contains tryptophan (a precursor to serotonin) is going to aid your ability to relax. Tryptophan can be found in lots of different foods and drinks, such as vegetable soup, dark chocolate, spinach and various herbal teas. You can also get it in milk but, as I'm not an advocate of consuming dairy products, I don't recommend drinking milk to get tryptophan. There are far healthier ways of getting the tryptophan into your diet.

I strongly suggest decreasing and – eventually – eliminating tea and coffee consumption: both of those are diuretics, which takes water out of your blood – the exact opposite of what we are trying to do! In addition, caffeine is a neurotoxin; in other words, it's toxic to your nervous system.

Being dehydrated definitely has an impact on your ability to relax and your ability to sleep at night. So, instead, *increase* your water intake: drink two to four litres (depending on your level of activity) of good quality pure filtered water. That's going to hydrate your body nicely and it will definitely aid your ability to relax and sleep at night. Chapter 2 covered water intake and recommendations in detail.

## Exercise

There are lots of different exercises that will aid your relaxation – Pilates, yoga, tai chi, etc. These are all very good and will aid relaxation, increase flexibility and general feelings of wellbeing. Pilates is an exercise that I've done for a long time myself – the best part of 20 years– and I find it very useful; it's something I recommend to a lot of my patients and coaching clients as well.

Yoga is something that I do periodically; when I go on meditation retreats, I'll do a lot of yoga, so I definitely advocate that.

Tai chi is something I've been interested for a long time and recently started doing; there are definite health benefits. Several of my private clients have done it for years and they have said it is very good for relaxation and I have to agree with them as I find it very calming.

However, the key to cracking the 'exercise' regime is to find an activity that *you enjoy doing* – so you'll stick to doing it. To get benefit it's crucial to do your exercise – whatever it is – consistently. If that means walking then go for a walk once (or more!) each day; or swimming, dancing, running, the gym. Whatever it is, make sure that you enjoy doing it, otherwise you will not do it consistently.

When you ***"get to"*** do an activity (rather than feeling like you ***"must do"*** or ***"should do"*** the activity) it feels very different! 'Getting to do something' is about choice and about enjoyment rather than the negative feeling a "must do" brings up.

Cardiovascular exercise is really important and resistance work of some kind is essential too, which we touched on in an earlier chapter. So when we do some exercise – whatever the exercise is – that is going to aid your ability to relax in the evening, just by getting the body moving. I cannot stress how critical it is to exercise – regularly – and find an exercise that you really enjoy doing.

## PUTTING IT ALL TOGETHER

It's not rocket science this thing! Keep it simple.

People are very prone to over-complicating most situations in life, so let's make it really, really simple. For *each* of the sections we have covered so far – mindset, nutrition and exercise – pick just one strategy. One mindset strategy (for example gratitude or intention); one nutrition strategy (say, increasing your water intake); one exercise strategy (going for a walk or going for a swim). Choose something that you get to do; so you will love doing it and you will do it consistently.

# CHAPTER SUMMARY

## Key Learning # 1: Causes of Exhaustion

Earlier in the chapter and section 1 we looked at the links between exhaustion and not sleeping; all of these related to the stress response and the release of stress hormones in your body. Then we looked at four reasons for exhaustion:

- **Insomnia** – this is a vicious cycle as it all feeds into, or exacerbates, the stress response

- **Anxiety** – feelings of anxiety will most likely lead to difficulty sleeping or insomnia, further contributing to exhaustion

- **Irrational fears** – again, this perpetuates the chronic stress response that's going on in the body when we are stressed out and exhausted; that stress response increases adrenaline in the body, decreases serotonin, increases anxiety, increases fear, decreases concentration and decreases short-term memory

- **Lack of time off**- again, this is another one that perpetuates the whole cycle.

## Key Learning # 2: Relax Better

To be able to relax better, you need to do three things, eat, move, and think on purpose:

- **Eat on purpose** – eating the right food and the right drink at the right time
- **Move on purpose** – movement is an essential nutrient for the brain, it powers up the brain and the body
- **Think on purpose** – a positive mindset is essential for health and wellbeing and rest and relaxation.

## Key Learning # 3: Sleep Like a Baby

We talked about how to sleep like a baby and how this had three main components: mindset, nutrition, and exercise. We ended the chapter with the task of picking one strategy from each element – and making a start on your move to a more healthy life style.

## *MY LEARNINGS & NEW COMMITMENTS*

_____

_____

_____

_____

_____

_____

_____

_____

_____

_____

_____

_____

_____

_____

_____

_____

_____

_____

_____

_____

# Conclusion

Let's bring it all together now. In this book we've explored how eating, moving and thinking on purpose can transform many areas of your life. As seen in the various case studies and testimonials there are a diverse range of clients who have benefitted from the Total Health Transformation system.

Whether you lack confidence in yourself; fear putting yourself out there to promote your business; you want to get in the best shape of your life for your wedding day or you want to get some pain relief from severe arthritis - Total Health Transformation is definitely for you.

We analyse how you currently do things, what your goals are; then we work together to turn your life around and quickly move you from where you are to where you want to be in record time!

The solution to the problems of demotivation, lack of energy, and poor health is the Total Health

Transformation Programme. As you have seen demonstrated throughout this book, the 3 parts to the system are all very much inter-connected and if any part is absent then the result is less than perfect! Just to recap those 3 parts are:

- **Eat on purpose**
- **Move on purpose**
- **Think on purpose**

## Eat on Purpose

It's vital to focus on foods that enhance the feelings of calm, peace and well-being; this will aid your quality of meditation, your ability to meditate and your ability to relax – which allows you to meditate well.

Eat plenty of vegetables and fruits – an easy way to get lots of vegetables and fruits into your body is by making homemade soups, juices and smoothies. Drink herbal teas and just eat lots of good quality organic fruits as well.

We also talked about decreasing your use of stimulants, so decrease your intake of teas and coffees: that will aid your meditation. Finally, increase your water intake as this will also aid your meditation practice.

## Move on Purpose

For some people, going for a walk can be a good form of meditation. One thing is for sure though: it's imperative to get your body moving, as that will aid your ability to relax and this, in turn, will improve your quality of meditation.

Regular exercise is crucial to the success of the Total Health Transformation programme. It's so important to implement a regular exercise regime into your life

Having regular chiropractic check-ups will help to realign your spine, so your brain and your body can 'communicate better.' We saw in an earlier chapter how this reconnects the brain to the body and allows the signals between different elements of your body to be more effective – so this will in turn allow you to sit more comfortably, and you'll be able to relax much better when you meditate.

The chiropractic adjustment will increase proprioception (your body's ability to be aware of itself in space) and decrease nociception (your sensory nervous system's response to certain harmful or potentially harmful stimuli). What this means, ultimately, is the bodies increased awareness of itself heightens all sensations; the decreased nociception lowers the sensitivity of pain receptors and pain.

## Think on Purpose

Once you learn how to master your emotions then you will begin to master your life. This is why we spend a long time focusing on mindset on the programme.

Strategies including Meditation, EFT and Sedona Method are just a handful of the tools we use to help you master your mind.

As I'm sure you can appreciate, the eating and moving parts of the system have a big impact on how well you can think on purpose. As mentioned in earlier chapters, lots of different foods will release serotonin and dopamine into your body, into your bloodstream; these will help make you feel relaxed yet focused and productive.

## Final Thoughts...

I've been in the healing arts for over 20 years and during that time and it's been my absolute pleasure to have been able to help so many people on their journey to optimal health and wellness. My vision for Total Health Transformation is to create a worldwide movement of people that are educated, inspired and empowered to transform their health and the health of their families and communities. We want to directly and indirectly have a transformational affect on the health at least 10 Million people worldwide. I would be honoured if you would help me share the message with those you care about. All the best!

# Your Next Steps...

Congratulations if you have made it here. You are already an exceptional individual – most people don't read books all the way to the end!

In this book I've done my best to map out the Total Health Transformation System that has helped hundreds of people transform their health. Now it's up to you to use this information and make it work for you.

## HOW TO GET IN TOUCH...

You can email me personally at **danny@dannyscahill.com**

We have a range of products and services all designed to help you achieve Optimal Health and Wellbeing. We offer workshops, coaching programmes (corporate and personal coaching), consultancies, keynotes and more. Get in touch and let us know how we can serve you best.

To Your Health, Wealth & Happiness,

*Dr Danny Scahill*

Dr Danny Scahill DC
Chiropractor & Peak Performance Expert

# About The Author

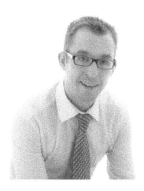

Dr Danny Scahill has been in the healing arts for over 20 years and in that time he has helped 1000's of people achieve Health Transformation. He is a Doctor of Chiropractic, Health & Wellness Expert and a Peak Performance Coach. This book "Total Health Transformation – The Proven System to Unlock Limitless Energy, Motivation & Health" is the culmination of over 20 years of Dr Scahill's experience in helping his patients and clients achieve a lifetime of Health and Wellness.

Through his Total Health Transformation Coaching programmes, Events, Podcasts, Articles and blog posts

Dr Danny continues to spread his message across the world – If you want to be truly Healthy you must Eat Move and Think On Purpose – with that purpose being Optimal Health.

Dr Danny Scahill is a captivating speaker and trainer that keeps people on the edge of their seats. He is very passionate about helping his audiences experience a health breakthrough. Having over came physical injury and depression at the age of 15, it was those experiences that inspired him to create the Total Health Transformation programmes years later.

Having already made a significant difference in the lives of many people around the world, Dr Danny Scahill looks forward to educating, inspiring and empowering millions more people to make better health choices so that they can live the lives they desire.

Milton Keynes UK
Ingram Content Group UK Ltd.
UKHW010653170124
436175UK00001B/7

9 780994 594